PHYSIOLOGY OF PURPOSE

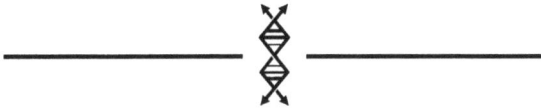

BRIAN BETANCOURT

ISBN:
eBook: 978-1-960346-80-3
Hardback: 978-1-960346-81-0
Paperback: 978-1-960346-82-7

\\\ AUTHORSUNITE

DEDICATION

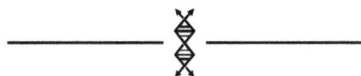

For those who forgot they could move—
and for those who are ready to remember.

ACKNOWLEDGMENTS

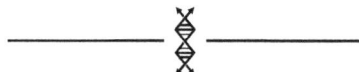

I owe this book to the people who helped shape the person behind it. This project wasn't built in isolation—it was built through years of mentorship, guidance, friendship, challenge, and love.

To **Jesus Gallo** and **Ed Downs**: You both made me see things in a whole new light. Your wisdom and perspective opened doors I didn't know were there.

To Juan Carlos Faraldo: Without knowing it, you inspired the first steps.
Watching you coach athletes with such precision and presence showed me what mastery could look like.
You led me to Gallo and set me on the path.

To Carlos Sainz: For teaching me how to grapple. For welcoming me and my wife when no adults were being taught. For shaping me into someone far more capable than I appear. Your guidance lives in every movement I trust.

To **Felix Flores**: Thank you for showing me the ropes in graduate school. You helped me navigate a world that could've easily overwhelmed me.

To **Charmaine DeFrancesco**: Your teaching forever changed the way I think about motor learning and skill development. You gave me a language for what I intuitively believed.

To **Bianca Leason**: Thank you for being the voice of reason. You've been more than a friend; you've been a coach, a mirror, and a guide.

To **Erwan Le Corre**: Thank you for creating MovNat and for helping me find language and structure for what I was trying to build on my own. Your work gave mine a home.

To my **wife, Stephanie**: You make me the luckiest man alive. Thank you for your patience, belief, and strength.

To my **parents**: Thank you for providing me with a solid foundation. You taught me resilience, creativity, and how to think for myself.

To my **brother, Jon**: You've always been my favorite grumpy sparring partner.

To every mentor, every coach, and every training partner who helped me grow: you left fingerprints on this work, whether you know it or not.

FOREWORD

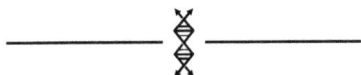

Human beings did not invent movement. Movement invented us. Long before we formed theories about physiology or wrote systems of training, the body already knew what to do: adapt, survive, evolve, and express capability through the intelligent orchestration of its own tissues and signals. My life's work has been an attempt to return to that fundamental truth — to help people remember that movement is not an optional activity but the original language of the human organism.

This book stands firmly inside that truth.

Physiology of Purpose is not another manual of exercises, nor a collection of motivational slogans dressed up as science. It is a map, one that reveals how deeply movement, perception, and physiology are intertwined. Brian Betancourt has done something rare here: he has written about the human body with both scientific rigor and lived understanding. He speaks with clarity, not complexity. He explains without diluting. And he respects the organism rather than reducing it to isolated parts.

Brian and I share a common conviction: capability is not built in controlled environments or through compartmentalized training. It emerges from the conversation between the nervous system and the real world; from uncertainty, pressure, and adaptation. Movement is not performance for its own sake. Movement is self-discovery. It is how the body learns trust, and how the mind learns truth.

Across these chapters, Brian brings that reality to the forefront. He shows how energy systems, neural circuits, sensory pathways, and emotional states work together as a single integrated intelligence. And he shows how our modern lifestyles, while convenient, often sever us from the very mechanisms that make us strong, resilient, and fully human.

There is something else in these pages that deserves to be acknowledged. Beneath the science and narrative runs a deeper message: that movement is a return. A return to capability. A return to presence. A return to the biological wisdom that shaped us long before we shaped anything in return. This is not nostalgia for a lost past; it is a recognition of what remains true, regardless of the era we live in.

I recognize the sincerity in Brian's work. I recognize the discipline it took to connect theory with lived practice. And I recognize his desire to give readers more than information, to give them orientation. Not the kind that tells you what to do, but the kind that changes the way you perceive what your body already knows.

If you read this book with attention, you will not finish it as the same mover you were when you began. You will understand your body more deeply, not as a machine to manage, but as a coordinated, adaptive, self-refining system. You will understand your nervous system as the command center of capability. And you may even recover a sense of trust in yourself that you thought was gone or unreachable.

Purpose is not an abstraction. It is something the body expresses before the mind ever defines it. That is the insight at the heart of this book, and why I am glad to see it in the world.

— Erwan Le Corre
Founder of MovNat
Founder of BreathHoldWork®

TABLE OF CONTENTS

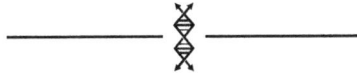

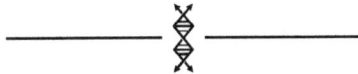

MY STORY

When I was a kid, I moved without a second thought. Basketball games in the driveway. Manhunt with the neighbors. Karate classes.

Long, aimless bike rides with my dad until the world blurred around us.

Movement was play. Movement was life.

But as I got older, life shifted.
In high school, after suffering an injury and experiencing academic setbacks, my dream of playing collegiate sports faded.

I found a new obsession: music. Jazz guitar became my world. I played for hours a day, hunched over, lost in sound instead of space. I ate whatever was fast and easy. I practiced until my fingers bled.

And I sat—more than I had ever sat in my life.

Then came the wake-up call: high cholesterol.

In my twenties.

My doctor gave me a choice: medication or movement.
I chose movement.
Bodybuilding.com became my Bible. I recruited a few friends,
joined a gym, and for years, we trained like machines. Split
routines. Protein shakes. Muscle groups by the day of the
week. It worked—for a while. But something still felt hollow.

I left music behind and tried to pivot toward physical therapy,
but university red tape blocked me.
Too many music credits. Not enough of the "right" ones.
So I took a course on Exercise Physiology instead.

And everything changed.

From the first lecture, I knew: *this is what I want to do for the
rest of my life.* I dove in headfirst, studying performance, energy
systems, and recovery. That same year, I took on a project to
design a strength and conditioning program for MMA fighters.
Research led me to a facility called South Miami Sports Performance. I showed up uninvited, asked to intern, and a week
later, I was hired. Functional training became my new religion.

But the real shift came years later, after working with both
athletes and clinical populations. I trained everyone from
youth competitors to people with heart disease, type 2
diabetes, and obesity. I saw both sides of the spectrum—and
still, something was missing.

Then came 2020, when the world shut down.
Gyms closed. Clients disappeared. And I found myself trying
to write a free e-book to help people move better at home. I
scribbled down ideas about locomotion, lifting, self-defense—
things I felt everyone should know. But something wasn't
clicking.

One night, while scrolling YouTube in bed, I found a podcast with **Erwan Le Corre**. Someone asked him: *"What is natural movement?"* He answered, *"Have you ever seen an out-of-shape eagle? Or an out-of-shape fish? You don't—unless they're in a zoo."*

Then he said, *"We're in a zoo."*

That was it.
I got out of bed, walked to my desk, and started reading everything I could find.
I downloaded the pages that didn't make it into his book. I devoured them.
And I remember walking up to my wife and saying, *"I need to do this certification."*

I signed up for MovNat L1 and L2.
October 2020.
And I never looked back.

For the first time, everything clicked.
I wasn't just studying physiology.
I was feeling it.
Living it.
Breathing it.
Trusting it.

Natural movement didn't replace my scientific understanding.
It deepened it, helping me connect the dots that the textbooks left out.
It made me see the body not just as a system of muscles and enzymes, but as a dynamic intelligence—always listening, always adapting.

This book isn't a manual.
It's a map.
A way back to something we were never meant to lose.

Movement isn't something you "work out" to earn.
It's something you remember.
It's something you are.

You don't need to be an athlete.
You don't need to be young.
You just need to move—because that's where the truth lives.
That's where purpose begins.

You were made for this.
You always have been.

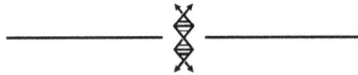

YOU FORGOT HOW TO MOVE

You were born to move.
Before you could speak, you could crawl, roll, balance, climb, squat, and reach.
Movement was your first language.

You didn't study it.
You didn't need to be taught.

You *solved* movement, moment by moment:

- You found ways to lift your head.
- You explored gravity by falling.
- You discovered reaching, standing, and climbing.

Every solution built a body.
Every body built a brain.

Somewhere along the way, you forgot.

You stopped crawling.
You stopped climbing.
You stopped trusting movement.

Not because you got lazy.
Not because you lost discipline.
But because the world around you stopped asking for it.

We engineered comfort.
We erased necessity.
We replaced adventure with schedules and exploration with workouts.

Movement became something you "have to do" instead of something you *are*.

But here's the truth:

- Movement isn't fitness.
- Movement isn't optional.
- Movement is **you.**

You don't need a new body.
You need a new relationship with the one you've had your whole life.

This book is your invitation to remember.

It's not a program.
It's not a challenge.
It's a map back to the beginning that you never actually lost.

You were born capable.

Let's help you remember. This isn't a return to fitness.

It's a return to remembrance.

And movement is the way back.

The pages ahead won't give you hacks or reps.

They'll show you how your body already knows the way.

Through energy.

Through nerves.

Through memory and breath and movement reborn.

CHAPTER 1

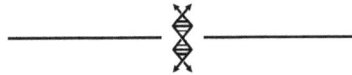

THE BODY'S ENERGY CODE

Why You Move the Way You Move (and Why It Matters)

He doesn't know how close they are.
He just knows they're coming.

A low growl from behind. Then another. Then, silence louder than any roar.

He runs.

Not gracefully. Not tactically. Not like an action hero. Just total, primal escape driven by instinct, environment, and whatever fuel his body can burn.

His arms pump harder than they need to. His legs over-extend. He barely blinks.
He doesn't look at the ground—he trusts it.

He doesn't feel the pain—he ignores it.
He doesn't think—he moves.

Roots. Branches. Slopes. Grit. Sweat.
He isn't navigating. He is surviving.

In this moment, every system in his body surges to keep him alive.

What Is Physiology—and Why Does It Matter?

Movement happens fast.
Physiology explains **how**.

Not to dissect it.
Not to reduce it.
But to understand the **miracle** that just unfolded inside your body.

Physiology is not just the study of the body—
It's our human attempt to describe the **orchestration of life**.

Like music theory emerged to explain the beauty of sound, physiology emerged to reveal the wonder of **existence in motion**.

It's an imperfect language trying to describe perfect complexity.

It's our way of saying, *"This is how the body sings when it runs, lifts, breathes, heals, and evolves."*

And What About Exercise Physiology?

Exercise physiology zooms in on moments like this—
the sprint, the climb, the fall, the rise—
and asks:

- What systems are working?
- How do they talk to one another?
- What is the purpose of fatigue, of effort, of adaptation?

And more importantly:

- How does movement make us more **resilient**, more **capable**, more **human**?

It's not just about physical fitness.
It's about survival.
It's about **becoming**.

Now that you've seen the runner run for his life,
Let's look under the surface.
Let's listen to the **orchestra playing inside him**.

Because the story you just read wasn't just about willpower.
That was **physiology**.

A Brief History of Physiology

What is Physiology?

Physiology is the scientific study of how living systems function. It asks: What keeps us alive? How do organs, tissues, and cells work together?

Ancient Roots

The origins of physiology trace back to Greek physicians Hippocrates (c. 400 BCE) and Galen (c. 200 CE), who studied bodily function through observation and dissection.

Scientific Revolution

In the 17th century, English doctor William Harvey discovered blood circulation, marking a significant shift toward evidence-based study.

Modern Physiology

The 19th century saw breakthroughs in cellular function, muscle contraction, and nerve signaling. Physiology became a formalized scientific discipline, integrated into medicine and biology.

Today, physiology is the foundation of medical science, helping us understand health, disease, performance, and adaptation.

A Brief History of Exercise Physiology

What is Exercise Physiology?

It's the study of how the body responds and adapts to movement, physical stress, and training. It explores energy production, muscle function, cardiovascular response, recovery, and other related topics.

Early 20th Century

Swedish scientist Per-Olof Åstrand and the Harvard Fatigue Laboratory (1927–1947) pioneered the empirical study of human performance and fatigue

Mid-century Boom

As sports and military training matured, so did research into VO_2 max, lactate, endurance, and strength adaptations.

Modern Era

The rise of elite athletics, fitness industries, and rehabilitation sciences has transformed exercise physiology into a global, multi-billion-dollar field.

Today, exercise physiology is applied in sports performance, chronic disease prevention physical therapy, and human optimization. It's not just about athletes, but understanding the movement that sustains life.

The Bioenergetic Orchestra: Fueling Movement

The wolves growl.
Your body moves before your mind has time to catch up.
Deep inside, a symphony begins.

So what exactly happens during that sprint?

To understand it, we need to look beneath muscles, beyond instinct, and into the biological engines that power movement itself.

ATP-PC System: The First Strike

The first system to activate during explosive effort is the **ATP-PC system** , your body's short-burst energy engine.

Buried inside every muscle fiber is a reserve of raw energy, **adenosine triphosphate** (ATP) and **phosphocreatine**, waiting for moments like this.

No planning.
No permission.
Just explosive action.

This system fuels the first leap off the ground, the first desperate strides across uneven earth.
It is short-lived, but in those first seconds, it is everything.

ATP-PC is the starter pistol of survival.

Glycolysis: The Fast Rhythm

As your ATP stores deplete, **glycolysis** kicks in, rapidly breaking down glucose to produce energy and fuel continued effort.

Glucose is broken down rapidly, yielding energy and the byproduct **lactate**.
Not as waste, but as a strategic pivot to keep you moving when oxygen can't keep up.

It's imperfect, frantic, and loud—but it's what keeps your feet flying forward and your mind sharp under pressure.

Glycolysis is the drumline of urgency.

The Lactate Shuttle: Adaptation in Motion

As lactate accumulates, your body adjusts by recycling it, utilizing the lactate shuttle to energize other tissues and maintain performance. **Lactate**, long misunderstood, becomes a courier of survival:

Fueling your heart.
Feeding your slow-twitch fibers.
Routing itself to the liver for transformation.

This isn't breakdown.
It's redistribution.

Your body moves resources, buys time, and extends your capacity in times of stress.

The lactate shuttle is the improvisation keeping the melody alive.

The Cori Cycle: Recycling the Song

As you move, the **Cori cycle** quietly converts lactate into glucose, recycling fuel through the liver to support ongoing exertion. It captures the excess lactate circulating through your blood and converts it back into usable glucose.

The **Cori cycle** doesn't move fast.
It's the slow, steady bassline behind the frantic front that restores fuel.

You don't just burn through resources.
You *regenerate* as you move.

The Cori cycle is the bass pulse keeping the orchestra grounded.

Fatty Acid Oxidation: The Endurance Engine

For longer efforts, the body shifts to **fatty acid oxidation**, a slower and more sustainable system that converts fat into usable energy.

Fatty acid oxidation turns fat into energy.

Quietly, dependently, relentlessly.

It's not made for sprinting.
It's made for survival across hours, landscapes, and life itself.

Fatty acid oxidation is the enduring hum of persistence.

How the Bioenergetic Orchestra Comes Together

These systems don't engage one after the other like dominoes. They overlap, interconnect, and communicate as needed.

1. ATP-PC fires the starting shot.

2. Glycolysis surges to carry the next moments.

3. The lactate shuttle and Cori cycle manage resources in real time.

4. Fatty acid oxidation builds the foundational endurance that sustains the entire effort.

They trade the lead like musicians in a jazz quartet—sometimes soloing, other times supporting, but always playing the same music:

Keep you moving.
Keep you capable.
Keep you alive.

No single fuel source or system powers our movement. Its crescendos burst from an orchestra trained through epochs of evolution, waiting for your next move.

And it plays whether you notice or not.

The Hormonal Orchestra: Conducting Readiness and Recovery

Your legs drive forward.
Your chest tightens.
But inside your body, another section of the orchestra rises—louder now, sharper now—guiding every next move.

Cortisol: The Early Call to Action

Cortisol is the body's primary readiness hormone—mobilizing fuel, heightening focus, and preparing you for intense action.

Often misunderstood as a "stress hormone," cortisol's real role is **readiness**.

It liberates fuel, sharpening your system for action:

- Mobilizing glucose from the liver
- Redirecting blood flow to muscles
- Preparing the mind for quick, decisive movement

It doesn't cause panic.
It **coordinates precision** under pressure.

> **Cortisol is the drummer, setting the pace before the first note of escape is even played.**

Glucagon: The Fuel Liberator

Glucagon raises blood sugar by signaling the liver to release stored glucose, ensuring muscles have fuel when intensity rises.

It works to:

- Raise blood sugar
- Ensure glucose is available where it matters most: the working muscles

Glucagon doesn't drive movement directly.
It makes sure the engines never run dry.

> **Glucagon is the bass drum—steady, reliable, unseen but essential.**

Insulin: The Strategic Withdrawal

During high-intensity movement, insulin suppresses its usual role, thereby delaying energy storage and keeping fuel available for action.

When survival is at stake, the body knows:

- Storing energy can wait.
- Using energy is the priority.

Later, when the threat passes, insulin will return, guiding nutrients back into cells, rebuilding what was broken, replenishing what was spent.

Insulin is the muted brass section—silent during the surge, swelling powerfully when the recovery begins.

IGF-1: The Architect Waiting in the Wings

IGF-1 supports recovery and adaptation, triggering muscle repair and growth in response to mechanical and metabolic stress.

Released in response to mechanical stress, metabolic challenge, and hormonal shifts, IGF-1:

- Triggers muscle repair
- Signals mitochondrial growth
- Prepares tissues not just to heal, but to come back stronger

It's not urgent.
It's inevitable.

If you survive the sprint, **IGF-1 ensures you emerge better prepared for the next one.**

> **IGF-1 is the hidden melody, the architect sketching the plans for a stronger, faster future, long before the dust settles.**

Adrenaline and Noradrenaline: The Sharp Strike

Adrenaline and noradrenaline surge during peak intensity, elevating heart rate, expanding airways, and sharpening reaction time.

- Increasing heart rate
- Dilating airways
- Heightening alertness and reaction time

These catecholamines sharpen every edge of your survival.

Where cortisol sets the drumbeat, adrenaline **spikes the cymbal**—flashing, urgent, unmistakable.

> **Adrenaline is the clash that makes every system pay attention.**

How the Hormonal Orchestra Comes Together

These hormones don't act alone.
They don't shout over each other.

They **listen, adjust, and time their entries perfectly** based on your body's needs:

- Cortisol leads the opening call to action.
- Glucagon liberates the fuel.
- Adrenaline strikes sharply to heighten the reaction.
- Insulin steps aside until the crisis ends, then reclaims order.
- IGF-1 watches from the wings, ready to build after the battle.

This isn't random chemistry.
It's a conversation.
An old language your body speaks fluently—refined not for ease, but for capability.

When you move, you don't just burn calories.
You awaken systems older than fear, older than memory—systems that know how to keep you alive, and make you stronger.

Movement calls the orchestra to life.
And your hormones conduct the rhythm between effort and evolution.

The Circulatory Orchestra: Moving Life Through the System

Your feet tear across the ground.
Your heart pounds inside your chest.
But this isn't panic.
This is precision.

Movement doesn't just demand effort.
It demands flow.
And your circulatory system answers with a performance older than memory.

The Heart: The Relentless Conductor

The heart pumps oxygen-rich blood to working muscles, increasing its rate to meet the metabolic demands of movement.

Every beat is a command:

- Deliver oxygen
- Move nutrients
- Sweep away waste
- Support the systems that support survival

As movement intensifies, the heart speeds its rhythm, matching demand with delivery, second by second.

The heart is the conductor that never leaves the podium.
It accelerates, decelerates, and orchestrates—without hesitation.

And it does so not once, not twice, but tens of thousands of times a day.

Not because it's forced.
Because it's built for it.

The Blood Vessels: The Dynamic Highways

Blood vessels dynamically dilate and constrict to regulate blood flow, delivering oxygen and clearing waste at every level.

- Arteries open wider to speed oxygen to where it's needed most.
- Veins contract and push blood back to the heart, aided by the squeeze of working muscles.
- Tiny capillaries expand at the edges, exchanging fuel for waste with breathtaking efficiency.

They are not rigid pipes.
They are **dynamic, reactive highways**—adapting every moment to keep the orchestra in tune.

The blood vessels are the flexible pathways that let energy move exactly where it's needed, exactly when it's needed.

Capillary Exchange: The Trade at the Edge

Capillaries are where fuel and waste trade hands, exchanging oxygen, carbon dioxide, glucose, and lactate at the cellular frontlines.

- Oxygen is offloaded into starving muscle cells.
- Carbon dioxide and lactate are picked up for removal.
- Glucose is delivered, fueling every contraction.

This exchange is invisible to the eye, but absolutely vital.

Without it, no system could survive more than a few seconds. With it, you endure.

> **Capillary exchange is the subtle process that enables effort.**

Venous Return: Movement Feeding Movement

Working muscles assist circulation—compressing veins to push blood back to the heart and sustain cardiac output.

Every step doesn't just cost energy.
It **creates flow**.

Movement doesn't just burn fuel.
It **creates life**.

> **Venous return is the hidden choreography—muscles and veins working together to keep you moving forward.**

How the Circulatory Orchestra Comes Together

None of these parts acts alone.

- The heart commands the tempo.
- The arteries adjust delivery routes.
- The capillaries trade resources at the frontlines.
- The veins carry the echoes of effort back home.

Movement is not only supported by circulation; it also activates, teaches, and strengthens it.

Without movement, the orchestra dulls.
Flow stagnates.
Function declines.

With movement, every beat, every vessel, every microscopic exchange becomes sharper, faster, more resilient.

You don't just survive because your heart beats.
You survive because your entire circulatory system works in harmony with you, rising to the occasion without complaint, without delay, without fail.

Movement is the conductor.
Flow is the music.

And your survival is the song.

The Cellular Orchestra: The Hidden Choir of Adaptation

The sprint ends.
The threat fades.
The world grows still.

But inside your body, the most profound movement is only beginning.

Because movement doesn't just demand.
It instructs.
It leaves behind a blueprint, a message written in molecular code:

"Adapt. Grow. Prepare for the next challenge."

And your cells listen.

Mitochondria: The Energy Architects

Physical stress signals your cells to grow more mitochondria, boosting your ability to produce energy over time. That stress sends a signal:

- Build more mitochondria.
- Make the engines stronger.
- Increase endurance at the very source.

Mitochondria are the microscopic power plants inside your muscles, your brain, and your heart.
They don't just produce energy-they expand your potential.

Every time you move under pressure, you aren't just getting tired.
You are increasing your biological capacity to meet future demands with greater strength, greater resilience, and greater grace.

> **Mitochondria are the builders of energy. Movement tells them to multiply.**

Heat Shock Proteins: The Guardians of Structure

Under stress, cells activate Heat Shock Proteins—molecular guardians that repair and protect vital proteins. Proteins stretch, bend, and sometimes falter.

But your body doesn't abandon them.
It deploys **Heat Shock Proteins (HSPs)**—microscopic repair crews who rush to refold, reinforce, and restore.

HSPs don't just fix what's broken.
They **upgrade your tolerance for stress**.

They make your cells harder to break the next time.

Heat Shock Proteins are the unseen guardians who ensure that survival isn't just about recovery—it's about reinforcement.

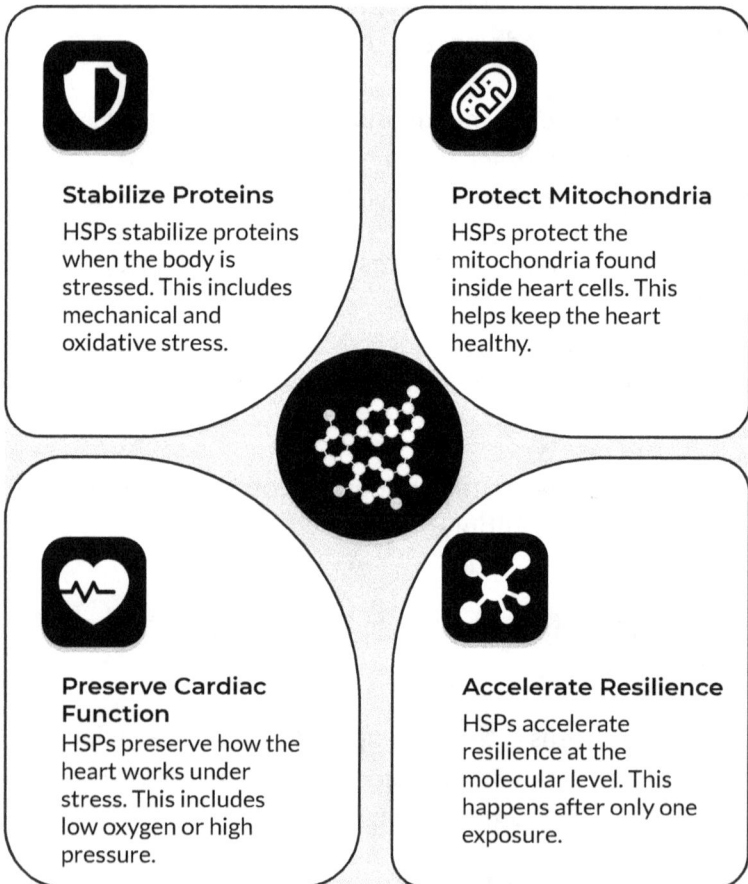

Stabilize Proteins

HSPs stabilize proteins when the body is stressed. This includes mechanical and oxidative stress.

Protect Mitochondria

HSPs protect the mitochondria found inside heart cells. This helps keep the heart healthy.

Preserve Cardiac Function

HSPs preserve how the heart works under stress. This includes low oxygen or high pressure.

Accelerate Resilience

HSPs accelerate resilience at the molecular level. This happens after only one exposure.

**HSP
Functions**

Neural Adaptation: The Brain Learns the Body

The nervous system learns through movement, refining speed, coordination, and reaction through repeated exposure.

This allows you to:

- Map this motion more efficiently.
- Reduce hesitation.
- Increase speed, accuracy, and instinct.

Neurons wire faster.
Pathways refine.
The nervous system doesn't just command the body—it evolves *with* it.

Every sprint, every stumble, every leap under pressure teaches your brain how to move better, faster, smarter.

Movement is education for the nervous system. Stress makes the lessons unforgettable.

How the Cellular Orchestra Comes Together

Deep beneath what you can see or feel, your cells are performing their own quiet symphony:

- Mitochondria are building new engines
- HSPs strengthening the architecture
- Neural circuits are wiring faster, cleaner, and stronger

This isn't passive healing.
It's active construction.
Movement doesn't just leave a memory.
It leaves a structure for a stronger life.

You don't just recover from effort.
You evolve because of it.

The Heart's Rapid Response

Your muscles adapt to stress over time.
But your heart?
It starts adapting **immediately**.

Even a single bout of intense movement triggers the production of **Heat Shock Proteins (HSPs)** inside cardiac tissue.

These HSPs:

+ **Stabilize proteins** under mechanical and oxidative stress

+ **Protect mitochondria** inside heart cells

+ **Preserve cardiac function** even under low-oxygen or high-pressure conditions

+ **Accelerate resilience** at the molecular level after just one exposure

This phenomenon, called **exercise preconditioning**, shows that **your heart becomes harder to break** from the very first challenge you give it.

Unlike skeletal muscle, which repairs and grows visibly, the heart adapts **quietly**, **efficiently**, and **early**–because it has no option to rest.

Every time you move with effort–whether sprinting, carrying, or climbing–you send a message to your heart: **"Prepare. Strengthen. Endure."**

And your heart listens.
Not weeks later.
Now.

Movement doesn't just build muscles.
It builds **a heart that's harder to break.**

The Symphony of Movement

Movement is not chaos.
It's not noise.
It's not random effort strung together by willpower.

It is **orchestration**— a coordinated, living performance where every system knows exactly when to rise, when to fall, and when to blend.

The Bioenergetic Orchestra

- ATP-PC strikes first, explosive and immediate.
- Glycolysis and lactate take the melody, urgent and imperfect but beautiful.
- The Lactate Shuttle and Cori Cycle manage the resources, keeping the tempo alive under strain.

- Fatty Acid Oxidation hums beneath it all, ready to carry the song across landscapes and lifetimes.

The Hormonal Orchestra

- Cortisol sets the rhythm, calling the body to action without hesitation.
- Glucagon liberates fuel like a steady bass drum.
- Insulin waits at the edge of the stage, ready to rebuild.
- IGF-1 sketches the blueprint for a stronger tomorrow.
- Adrenaline strikes sharp—urgency without panic.

The Circulatory Orchestra

- The heart commands, never missing a beat.
- Arteries, veins, and capillaries flex and adapt, moving life across the stage.
- Every step doesn't just burn energy—it circulates strength.

The Cellular Choir

- Mitochondria multiply, quietly preparing you for greater endurance.
- Heat shock proteins protect your internal structure, making you more resilient to breakage.
- Neural circuits wire new patterns faster and more fluently with every effort.

Together, They Play

No system alone could sustain you.
No single note could carry the song.

It's the *overlap*, the *adaptation*, the *elegance* of the systems moving together that allows you to survive, to thrive, and to evolve.

When you sprint, when you climb, when you crawl, when you carry—
You don't just use these systems.
You **activate them**.
You **refine them**.
You **expand them**.

Movement doesn't just reveal capability.

Movement creates it.

The True Meaning of Movement

Every time you move with purpose, you aren't just exercising.
You are **sending instructions deep into your biology**:

- Build better fuel systems.
- Strengthen your heart.
- Harden your cells.
- Sharpen your brain.
- Adapt faster next time.

You aren't just surviving movement.
You are becoming more capable because of it.

This Is the Physiology of Purpose.

Movement isn't optional.
Movement isn't supplemental.
Movement is the signal—the conductor—the language—
through which your body learns to thrive.

And it's happening whether you realize it or not.

The Physiology of Purpose

Move like it matters. Because inside you, it always does.

CHAPTER 2

———— ⚕ ————

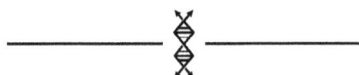

MOVEMENT MADE THE MIND

The Journey Begins: A Life Built Through Movement

He was born into a world he could not yet control.

The room was color, noise, blurred faces.
The body he occupied was not yet his own. Just a vessel of reflexes and flailing limbs—instincts firing in the dark.

But even then, movement had already begun to shape him.

The earliest wobbles of his arms, the reflexive kicks of his legs, the first uncoordinated attempts to reach a hand toward a voice— all of it sent ripples into the architecture of his brain.

When he learned to **crawl**, it wasn't just his body that moved forward. His brain stitched new circuits with every reach, every shift of weight, every tiny miscalculation corrected on the fly, building balance, coordination, spatial awareness, and confidence.

Movement taught the brain how to perceive the world and how to act within it.

It didn't happen by sitting still.
It happened by moving—fumbling, failing, adapting, succeeding.

As a child, the world expanded.

He climbed trees without fear, hung upside down from branches, and leapt from rocks to soft patches of earth below. He learned not by being told how to move, but by **experiencing how movement worked.**

A misstep taught him balance.

A slip taught him friction.

A leap taught him flight—and consequence.

Neurons fired and wired at a breathtaking pace.
His **cerebellum** made finer and finer adjustments.
His **sensory cortex** mapped the skin, joints, and limbs to an increasingly detailed understanding of the "self."
His **prefrontal cortex** began to predict, to plan, to imagine new ways to solve the problems his body encountered.

Movement didn't follow thought.
Movement taught thought how to exist.

Adolescence brought power and risk.

His movements became sharper, faster, and more complex. He ran trails, balanced on fallen trees, vaulted over obstacles without stopping to calculate.

The **basal ganglia** matured, smoothing his actions into seamless flows.
The **motor cortex** refined speed and efficiency.
The **emotional brain**—still raw—flooded him with adrenaline and ambition.

He learned, not always easily, that movement could be a way to test limits—or overreach them.

But always, movement sharpened the mind, revealing the edges of his capabilities and the cost of ignoring them.

Adulthood demanded more than strength.

It demanded adaptability.

He moved now not just for exploration, but for survival, for work, for others.
Heavy carries across fields.
Scrambling across unstable terrain.
Calm, deliberate movement under pressure.

The prefrontal cortex, once a blank canvas, now paints complex strategies in real time.
The cerebellum, once struggling to balance a crawling baby, now orchestrated micro-adjustments across hundreds of joints without conscious thought.

He wasn't *using* movement.
He was movement—refined, intuitive, capable.

And time marched forward still.

PHYSIOLOGY OF PURPOSE

He was no longer young.

The power of pure speed had faded.
But in its place: skill, fluidity, intelligence.

He moved differently now—less wasteful, more intentional.
Slow walking across uneven ground became a study in
subtlety.
Crawling, balancing, and climbing—all re-entered his life not as
childish games, but as necessary skills to keep mind and body
alive and well.

Beneath the surface, the **glymphatic system**—the brain's
cleansing river—flowed more effectively because of the
movement he still practiced.
Each session of mindful motion cleared debris from his brain,
refreshed his mind, and protected his memory.

Movement didn't just keep him strong.
It kept him sharp, awake, and connected.

From the first chaotic kicks of infancy to the graceful
problem-solving of older age, one truth never changed:

Movement built the brain.
Movement preserved the mind.
Movement taught him who he could become.

And in every stage of life, it was never just about muscles or
joints or skill.

It was about building the system that would carry him through
everything else.

But what is that system?

Let's look beneath the story, to the structures movement built, refined, and preserved.

The Brain Was Built for Movement

Long before language.
Long before planning.
Long before memory, tools, or culture—
there was movement.

Movement came first. Everything else—the mind, the memory, the story—followed.

And it was movement that shaped everything else.

When life first demanded survival on land, **the brain evolved not to think, but to move.**

Early neural structures developed to do one thing:

- Sense the environment
- React to threats
- Navigate terrain
- Find food
- Escape predators

Every neural innovation—from simple reflex arcs to complex decision-making—emerged because **moving well meant surviving longer.**

Before there was vision as we know it, there were light-sensitive patches to guide navigation.
Before there were emotions as we know them, there were primitive brain signals guiding *approach* or *avoidance*.

The first purpose of the brain was not to "know."
The first purpose of the brain was to "move."

Cognition, memory, language—all these gifts—came much later, layered atop a foundation of movement intelligence.

Even today, your most ancient brain structures—the **brainstem**, the **cerebellum**, the **basal ganglia**—are deeply intertwined with **movement control**.

And the sensory systems that define your interaction with the world—**vision, touch, balance, proprioception**—exist to serve **movement mastery** first, not abstract knowledge.

The ability to move through space created the need to map space.
Mapping space created the need to remember space.
Remembering space created the need to imagine new spaces.
And imagination gave birth to the mind as we know it.

In this way, **movement is not separate from intelligence**. Movement is the *ancestor* of intelligence.

You move, therefore you are.

Brainstem: The Foundation of Survival

What it is:
The **brainstem** sits at the base of your brain, connecting it directly to your spinal cord.
It is the brain's ancient root—a survival system forged before thought.

What it does:
It controls the basics—breathing, heart rate, blood pressure,

sleep-wake cycles, and reflexive postural adjustments.
It's where life-sustaining movement begins: keeping you
upright, breathing, alert, and ready.

The brainstem doesn't wait for
conscious thought.
It acts before you even know
you need it.

Brain stem

Why it matters:
Without a functioning
brainstem, movement isn't just
harder.
It's impossible.
Your very ability to be alive
and responsive depends on this hidden foundation—steady,
resilient, ever-present.

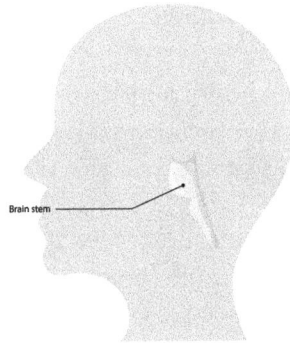

Movement practice, from simple standing balance to
breath-driven crawling, strengthens the brainstem's ability to
coordinate life itself.

Movement both arises from and strengthens the brainstem,
refining the core of your survival.

Cerebellum: The Architect of Precision

What it is:
The **cerebellum** is tucked under the back of your brain, behind
the brainstem.
It's small, but it houses over half the neurons in your entire
brain.

What it does:
It fine-tunes every motion:

- Smooths your movements
- Coordinates timing and sequencing
- Adjusts posture and balance
- Allows fluid transitions from one action to the next

If the brainstem keeps you alive, the cerebellum makes survival graceful.

From your first crawl to your most refined vault, the cerebellum is learning. Every movement that demands timing, sequencing, or adjustment is a gift of cerebellar refinement.

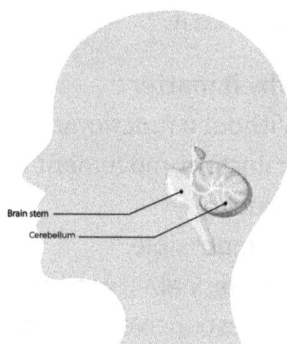

Brain stem

Cerebellum

Why it matters:
The cerebellum isn't just about movement elegance.
It's deeply tied to cognitive flexibility, emotional regulation, and learning.
Movement that challenges coordination doesn't just build elegance. It builds cognition.

Every time you balance on a beam, leap a gap, or adjust mid-fall, you are strengthening the part of your brain that teaches you how to adapt—not just in movement, but in life.

Basal Ganglia: The Engine of Skill and Habit

What it is:
The **basal ganglia** are a group of deep brain structures tucked under the cerebral cortex.

They act like a control center, refining voluntary movements and automating repeated patterns.

What it does:
When you first learn a new movement—crawling, balancing, vaulting—it feels awkward and deliberate.
But with repetition, the basal ganglia take over:

- Smoothing transitions
- Filtering unnecessary movements
- Turning conscious skills into automatic patterns

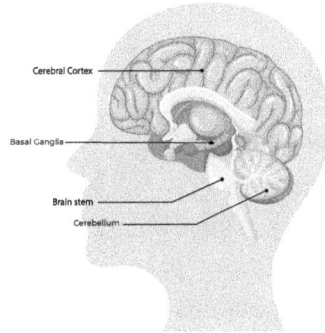

The basal ganglia allow you to move without thinking, freeing up your mind to focus elsewhere.

Why it matters:
Without the basal ganglia, every step would feel like the first, every climb like a brand-new challenge.

However, thanks to this ancient system, you can navigate complex environments with ease, precision, and efficiency.

> **Mastery isn't magic.**
> **It's the basal ganglia, turning effort into fluency.**
> **Repetition into readiness**

When you practice natural movement patterns—balancing, crawling, climbing—you aren't just building muscle memory. You are shaping deep neural pathways that automate competence.

Thalamus: The Gatekeeper of Sensation

What it is:
The **thalamus** sits deep in the center of the brain, acting as a relay station.

What it does:
Almost every sensory signal—touch, vision, balance, proprioception—passes through the thalamus before reaching higher processing centers.

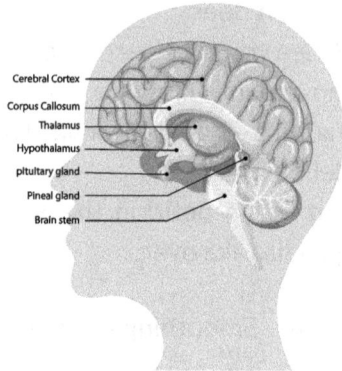

Cerebral Cortex
Corpus Callosum
Thalamus
Hypothalamus
pituitary gland
Pineal gland
Brain stem

It decides:

- What information gets through
- What gets prioritized
- What gets quieted

In a chaotic environment—running across uneven terrain, vaulting obstacles—the thalamus sorts and filters the flood of sensory input so you can stay focused and responsive.

Why it matters:
The thalamus protects your brain from overload.
It ensures that you feel what matters most when it matters most.

Training in natural movement—especially in complex, varied environments—sharpens the thalamic gate:
It teaches your brain to respond more quickly. To focus more sharply. To act more cleanly.

In a world of endless noise, the thalamus trains you to hear the signal.

Sensory Cortex: The Map of Your World

What it is:
The **sensory cortex** runs like a headband across the top of your brain, just behind the motor cortex.
It's where your brain receives and interprets sensory information from your body.

What it does:
Every time you touch the ground, feel the pull of gravity, and sense the texture of a tree branch under your hand, that data flows into the sensory cortex.

It builds:

- Maps of your body
- Awareness of your limbs in space (proprioception)
- Sensory memories that guide future movement

Without a clear sensory map, movement becomes clumsy, unsafe, and inefficient.

Why it matters:
When you crawl, balance, climb, or vault, you aren't just moving—you're refining the precision of your internal body map.

A sharper sensory cortex means:

- Faster reactions
- Better balance
- Greater adaptability

Movement sharpens perception.

Perception sharpens movement.

One teaches the other.

They grow together.

Every rock you scramble across, every branch you grasp, every stumble you recover from teaches your sensory cortex how to know the world—and yourself—more clearly.

Motor Cortex: The Origin of Intentional Action

What it is:
The **motor cortex** lies just in front of the sensory cortex.
It's the region that initiates voluntary movement.

What it does:
When you decide to step forward, leap, balance, or crawl—just like the hiker who fled through the forest, your motor cortex doesn't just move. It reacts. It plans. It commands. The motor cortex organizes the firing of neurons that tell muscles how to contract, when to contract, and in what sequence.

Just like the hiker who sprinted from wolves in Chapter 1, your motor cortex doesn't just move—it responds, plans, and recalibrates in real time.

Every shift in his stride, every leap over a fallen branch, every duck under a limb was initiated here—by a region of the brain translating raw urgency into precise, survival-driven action.

His escape wasn't mindless. It was the mind embodied— thought in motion.

It's where:

- Intention becomes motion
- Planning becomes execution
- Thought becomes action

Why it matters:
The motor cortex doesn't just command movement.
It adapts based on the movement challenges you face.

New, complex, real-world movements—balancing across a fallen tree, leaping a gap, pulling yourself over a ledge—force the motor cortex to grow sharper and stronger.

Movement challenges don't just reveal your brain's capacity. They expand it.

When you move into complex, variable environments, you forge a brain capable of not just reacting, but solving, adapting, and thriving under pressure.

Prefrontal Cortex: The Architect of Strategy and Meaning

What it is:
The **prefrontal cortex** sits at the very front of your brain—the most recently evolved, most human part of your mind.

What it does:
It plans.
It anticipates.
It imagines.

When you decide not just to leap but to *measure the risk* first—when you map the best path across a field of obstacles—when you pause to strategize instead of reacting mindlessly—that's your prefrontal cortex in action.

It governs:

- Foresight
- Decision-making
- Emotional regulation
- Moral judgment

In movement, the prefrontal cortex orchestrates *not just how you move*, but **why** you move.

Why it matters:
Without it, survival would be reactive and short-lived.
With it, survival becomes sustainable, and life becomes meaningful.

The more you move in ways that demand problem-solving— navigating uneven terrain, adapting your balance, choosing strategies on the fly—the more potent your prefrontal architecture becomes.

You aren't just refining motor skills. You're cultivating foresight.

Every complex movement is an act of planning, adaptation, and growth.
Movement refines the brain regions that define who you are.

Glymphatic System: The Brain's Cleansing River

What it is:
The **glymphatic system** is the brain's hidden cleaning mechanism.
It clears metabolic waste, toxins, and damaged proteins from neural tissue, primarily during deep sleep.

What it does:
When you move through your day—running, climbing, solving problems—your brain burns enormous amounts of energy.

This leaves behind byproducts—like amyloid proteins—that must be cleared to prevent cognitive decline, memory loss, and disease.

During quality sleep—especially after days rich with movement—the glymphatic system:

- Flushes waste
- Restores neural environments
- Protects long-term brain health

Movement during the day improves circulation, respiratory rhythms, and lymphatic drainage—all of which **optimize glymphatic function at night**.

Why it matters:
Without regular activation of this system, the brain literally clogs itself over time.
But with movement and sleep aligned, the brain renews itself—night after night, year after year.

Movement during the day is an investment.
Sleep is the dividend.
The glymphatic system cashes the check that keeps your
mind young.

Natural movement isn't just about surviving today.
It's about preserving the mind for tomorrow.

The Spine: Your Living Axis

Beneath the skin, beneath the breath, a column of motion
rises:
the spine.

Not a stiff rod.
Not a passive post.
A living axis built for freedom, for perception, for adaptability.

From infancy, the spine teaches the brain how to move:
Rolling builds segmentation.
Crawling refines coordination.
Climbing teaches extension and flexion in rhythm.

Each vertebra doesn't simply stack. It moves three-dimensio-
nally:
Flexion and extension.
Rotation.
Lateral shift.

Spinal joints are densely packed with proprioceptors and
mechanoreceptors that tell the brain:
Where am I?
How am I aligned?
How do I adjust?

A stiff spine is a silent spine.
A dynamic spine sings to the brain, constantly updating the sensory map of the self.

Freedom of spinal movement doesn't just support mobility. It supports cognition, awareness, and adaptability.

A supple spine = an adaptable mind.
From crawling infants to agile elders, spinal intelligence is movement intelligence made visible.

What Are Amyloid Proteins?

Amyloid proteins are fragments of larger proteins that, under normal conditions, are cleared away during brain maintenance (primarily during sleep).

When this process falters, these fragments accumulate and clump together, forming plaques that disrupt brain function—a hallmark of Alzheimer's disease and other types of dementia.

Regular movement enhances circulation, lymphatic drainage, and glymphatic function, all of which help prevent amyloid buildup.
Move well. Sleep well. Keep your mind clear.

What Is the Glymphatic System—and Why Was It "Hidden"?

The **glymphatic system** was only discovered in 2012. For decades, scientists had assumed that the brain lacked a lymphatic cleanup system, like the rest of the body.

But research uncovered a network of fluid channels that flush out waste during deep sleep, supported by glial cells—hence the name **"glymphatic"** (glial + lymphatic). Its late discovery is one reason why the impact of movement on brain detox wasn't fully understood until recently.

Astrocytes: The Hidden Architects of Memory and Metabolism

The neurons of the brain have long been likened to its electric stars, firing and always in motion.
But recent research reveals another force operating in the background, quieter but no less powerful: astrocytes.

These star-shaped glial cells form a vast network interwoven with neurons, not just supporting them but interacting with them, sensing their activity, and shaping their function. A single astrocyte can contact up to 2 million synapses. And when it does, it doesn't just listen, it learns.

Astrocytes do not generate action potentials. However, they communicate via **calcium signaling** and release **gliotransmitters** into synapses. This allows them to influence when and how neurons fire, subtly modulating the flow of information in the brain.

What does this mean for movement?

Everything.

Astrocytes form what neuroscientists now refer to as **tripartite synapses, three-part** junctions where the presynaptic neuron, the postsynaptic neuron, and an astrocyte all come together. These junctions are not just highways for electrical data; they are intersections where movement patterns, memories, and metabolic states converge.

Recent models suggest that astrocytes may act as a kind of **biological dense associative memory system**, enabling the brain to store vastly more information than neurons alone could manage. This memory isn't stored in electric spikes, but in the shifting **calcium patterns** and **gliotransmitter dynamics** of astrocyte networks.

The Brain's Movement Systems: A Symphony in Sections

While we've explored the brain piece by piece, your brain doesn't operate as a list of parts. It functions as a living ensemble—sections of a greater orchestra—where different regions collaborate to produce intelligent, adaptive movements.

Each cluster of structures contributes something vital:

The Survival System

Composed of the **brainstem, thalamus**, and parts of the **hypothalamus**, this system keeps you alive long before conscious thought begins.

It governs:

- Breathing
- Heart rate
- Arousal and sleep
- Reflexive posture and startle responses

This is your **a**lways-on network—quiet, steady, and utterly essential.
Before you move with skill, you survive by instinct.

The Motor System

Made up of the **motor cortex**, **cerebellum**, and **basal ganglia**, this system turns intention into action.

Together, they:

- Initiate movement (motor cortex)
- Refine timing and transitions (cerebellum)
- Automate patterns (basal ganglia)

This is the **movement engine** of your brain—balancing coordination, precision, and efficiency.

The Sensory System

Built from the **thalamus**, **sensory cortex**, and **proprioceptive pathways**, this system ensures your brain isn't flying blind.

It:

- Collects and filters environmental input
- Builds internal maps of your body in space
- Guides movement with real-time feedback

Without it, you would move clumsily, inefficiently—like swinging in the dark.

The Executive System

Centered in the **prefrontal cortex** and surrounding association areas, this system brings **foresight** to movement.

It handles:

- Planning and risk assessment
- Emotional regulation
- Multi-step problem-solving
- Goal-directed action

It's the reason a climber pauses to scan a rock face instead of rushing forward blindly.
It doesn't just move the body—it moves it with purpose.

The Emotional and Memory System (Limbic System)

Composed of the **hippocampus**, **amygdala**, and **cingulate cortex**, the limbic system gives meaning to movement.

It:

- Connects emotion to experience
- Associates movement with memory (pleasant or painful)
- Influences motivation and avoidance

This is why you remember the thrill of your first successful vault—or the fear of a near fall.

It's not just stored in muscle.
It's written in the emotional maps of your brain.

These systems do not compete. They coordinate.
They trade leadership.
They hand off responsibility mid-movement.

Together, they form a living architecture—a brain built not to sit still, but to solve the world through movement.

The Brain's GPS: How the Hippocampus Builds Space and Memory

The **hippocampus**, part of the limbic system, plays a dual role:

✦ *It maps space (so you know where you are).*

✦ *It encodes memories (so you know where you've been).* Movement—especially navigating uneven terrain, orienting toward landmarks, or solving spatial problems—directly stimulates hippocampal activity. Inactive people show faster hippocampal shrinkage with age. Movers preserve it—and with it, memory and direction.

The Brain on the Move: A Summary of Systems

System	Key Structures	Role in Movement
Survival System	Brainstem, Thalamus, Hypo-thalamus	Maintains vital functions: breath, heart rate, arousal, posture
Motor System	Motor Cortex, Cerebellum, Basal Ganglia	Initiates, refines, and automates skilled movement
Sensory System	Thalamus, Sensory Cortex, Propriocep-tors	Maps the body, filters environ-mental input, guides reactive adjustment
Executive System	Prefrontal Cortex, Association Areas	Plans actions, assesses risk, solves problems under pressure
Emotional/ Memory System	Hippocampus, Amygdala, Cingu-late Cortex	Attaches memory and emotion to movement; drives motivation and avoidance

The Brain as a Living Map: Integration Through Movement

The brain is not a collection of isolated parts.
It is a living map—dynamic, layered, woven together by every movement you make.

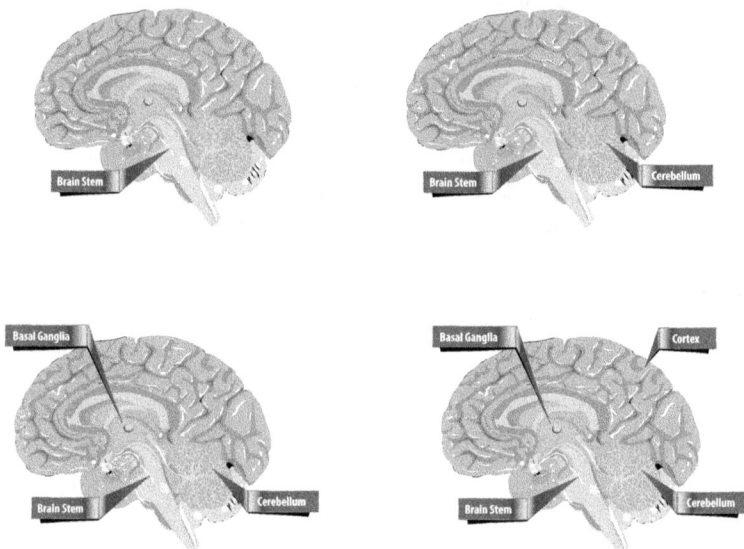

Neuroplasticity: Movement as Brain Remodeling

Neuroplasticity is your brain's ability to change itself—physically and functionally—in response to experience.

+ New skills forge new connections.

+ Repetition strengthens them.

+ Lack of use prunes them away. Natural movement challenges—balancing, crawling, navigating

> uncertainty—stimulate neuroplasticity in ways
> that seated learning cannot. *The body learns. The*
> *brain rewires.*

Each structure plays its role:

- The **brainstem** regulates essential functions such as breathing, standing, and alertness.

- The **cerebellum** refines your balance, your timing, and your fluidity.

- The **basal ganglia** automate your skills, transforming repetition into mastery.

- The **thalamus** filters the flood of sensation into signals that matter.

- The **sensory cortex** builds the map of your body and the world it moves through.

- The **motor cortex** translates thought into action, moment by moment.

- The **prefrontal cortex** plans, foresees, imagines, and chooses how you move and why.

- The **glymphatic system** protects the brain from decay, cleaning and renewing it through cycles of movement and rest.

However, these structures do not function independently. Not isolated instruments—but a living ensemble.

They are **an ensemble**—coordinating, learning, adapting, building you with every step, every reach, every leap into the unknown.

Movement isn't just output from this system.
Movement is what sculpts it.

- When a baby crawls toward a new sound, neurons wire pathways for exploration and curiosity.

- When a child climbs a tree, balances on a branch, and leaps to the ground, he strengthens circuits for prediction, correction, and resilience.

- When a young adult scrambles across a rugged trail, adapting to each unstable step, his brain becomes faster, wiser, and more robust.

- When an aging mover carries loads, balances on beams, and crawls across uneven surfaces, the brain retains its plasticity, sharpness, and vitality.

Why Movement Builds Cognitive Reserve

Cognitive reserve refers to the brain's capacity to resist age-related decline or injury by developing additional neural connections through challenges and learning. Active lifestyles, particularly those rich in movement complexity, are associated with a slower onset of dementia, even among individuals with a high amyloid burden. Each movement-rich day adds another brick to your neural fortress.

**Movement isn't something you do once the brain is ready.
Movement is how the brain becomes ready.**

It is how you develop perception.
It is how you build planning.
It is how you maintain memory, adaptability, and independence across the entire span of life.

Without movement, the ensemble falters.

The song begins to fade.

But with movement—deliberate, varied, challenging, joyful—
the brain stays alive.
It stays responsive.
It stays *human*.

Movement is not just a skill you keep.
It's a mind you preserve.

The Physiology of Purpose

Move like it matters.
Because inside you, it always does.

Movement makes the brain.
Movement refines the brain.
Movement preserves the brain.

Across every stage of life—
you move to become who you are meant to be.

CHAPTER 3

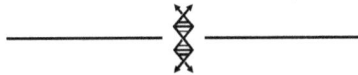

THE SENSORY
SYMPHONY

Falling Into Awareness

The sprint tore across the clearing.

His feet smashed against the uneven ground, lungs heaving,
eyes scanning for an opening—any opening—that might lead
him to safety.

Behind him, the predators gave chase.
The forest blurred into green and gold and shadow.
There was no time to think, only to move.

And then—
a misstep.

The ground, once solid, betrayed him.
His foot slid against slick leaves, throwing his balance
sideways.
In a heartbeat, the chase became a fall.

Time slowed.

Every system, trained through a lifetime of movement, surged forward—not to panic, but to perform.

Vestibular signals fired from deep within his inner ear—screaming of tilt, acceleration, and sudden danger to balance.

Proprioceptive signals surged from every joint and tendon—mapping limb position, recalibrating angles and pressure in real time.

Visual input narrowed and sharpened—catching the blur of earth rushing up, scanning slope, obstacles, angles.

Tactile feedback lit up his palms, forearms, and shins—readying him to feel, adjust, and absorb.

Interoceptive whispers stirred within—heart pounding, lungs flooding, muscles primed for impact or redirection.

Auditory signals caught the crack of leaves, the rumble of shifting ground, the soft signals of the world closing in.

And beneath it all, like a distant drumbeat, **nociceptive systems** braced—preparing neural circuits for pain, ready to survive impact if the landing went wrong.

But it didn't go wrong.

His body—trained through a lifetime of natural movement—knew what to do.

Instead of stiffening, he bent.

Instead of freezing, he flowed.

The slip became a tuck—
a shoulder leading the roll,
a hip swinging wide,
a foot sweeping around to find earth again.
He didn't stop the fall.

He shaped it.
He rolled.
He rose.
He ran—
not as a perfect machine,
but as a human being
whose senses had been trained
to solve the unthinkable
before thought could even begin.

This wasn't luck.
It wasn't instinct alone.

It was the quiet, powerful collaboration of the senses—
vestibular, proprioceptive, visual, tactile, interoceptive,
auditory, nociceptive—
all converging in a split-second of orchestration.

Movement didn't just happen.
It was awareness, becoming action.

The Sensory Orchestra: Movement's Invisible Guide

Long before thought, before strategy, before conscious
planning—
movement was guided by sensation.

The ability to survive, to navigate, to recover from a fall or a strike—
all depends on the senses working together, in real time, beneath awareness.

Your sensory systems are not passive observers.
They are active architects of action.

Every step, every leap, every dodge, every recovery—
is built on their silent conversation.

The human sensory system weaves seven major threads into one fabric of perception:

- **Vestibular**—sensing head position, gravity, acceleration
- **Proprioceptive**—mapping joint, limb, and body position internally
- **Visual**—scanning and predicting external threats and pathways
- **Auditory**—locating and reacting to sound cues in space
- **Tactile**—feeling surface, friction, contact, texture
- **Interoceptive**—sensing internal states (heart rate, breath, stress)
- **Nociceptive**—detecting potential harm and triggering a protective response

Each system gathers raw information.
But none act alone.

They integrate.
They compare.
They refine.

They orchestrate movement—before you even know you need it.

In the seconds it took the hiker to slip, roll, and rise,
all seven systems fired, collaborated, and adapted in real time—
not just responding, but solving.

This is the sensory orchestra.
This is movement before thought.
This is the beautiful, invisible guide that allows human beings not just to react to the world,
but to move through it with resilience, intelligence, and grace.

Vestibular and Proprioceptive Systems: Mapping Movement From Within

Vestibular System: The Balance Compass

What it is:
The vestibular system lives deep inside your inner ear.
It detects head position, rotation, acceleration, and the pull of gravity.

What it does:
Every time you tilt, spin, stumble, or even subtly shift posture, the vestibular system fires instantly.
It tells the rest of your body:

- Where "up" is
- How fast you're moving
- How sharply you're turning

- How your head's orientation relates to your body and the world

And it does all this before conscious thought arrives.

Why it matters:
The vestibular system is your internal gyroscope.
Without it, balance disintegrates.
Posture collapses.
Spatial orientation unravels.

When you train dynamic balance—walking beams, crawling across uneven ground, recovering from slips—you aren't just practicing skill.
You're sharpening your brain's ability to map the invisible forces of gravity and acceleration.

Balance isn't luck.
It's a continuous, quiet symphony of micro-signals—
played inside your skull,
conducted by the fluid in your inner ear,
and felt in every step you take.

How the Inner Ear Maps Movement

Tucked deep within the dense bones of your skull lies one of the most extraordinary pieces of biological engineering ever discovered:
The vestibular system.

Small. Almost hidden.
And yet, it allows you to:

✦ **Balance**

- **Coordinate**
- **Navigate**
- **Recover from falls**

—all without conscious thought.

It works through two powerful structures:

The Semicircular Canals: Rotation Sensors

*Three tiny, fluid-filled loops, each arranged at a right angle to the others. Together, they detect rotational movement in all three planes: **pitch, yaw, and roll.***

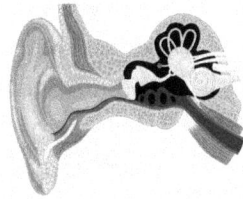

When you turn your head, fluid shifts inside the canals, bending delicate, hair-like sensors. These sensors fire nerve impulses that signal:

- *You are spinning.*
- *You are tilting.*
- *You are rotating.*

The Otolith Organs (Utricle and Saccule): Gravity and Acceleration Sensors

Flat membranes weighted with microscopic crystals—like tiny biological sandbags.
*These detect **linear acceleration** and **gravitational pull**.*

When you move forward, backward, up, down—or even tilt your head—

*the "ear stones" (**otoconia**) shift.*
They bend the sensory hairs beneath them, signaling:

- ✦ **You are moving forward.**
- ✦ **You are falling.**
- ✦ **You are upright—or you're not.**

Why This Matters

When you slip, jump, fall, or recover,
your vestibular system unleashes a cascade of precise,
rapid-fire signals—
giving your body the data it needs to act faster than
conscious thought.

Without these tiny structures working in harmony,
even standing still would feel like trying to balance on a
ship in a storm.

These systems aren't optional.
They're the invisible scaffolding of every movement you
make.

Proprioceptive System: The Internal Body Map

What it is:
The proprioceptive system is a web of sensors in your muscles,
tendons, and joints.
It builds a continuous, real-time map of your body's position
in space—no mirrors, no cameras, no conscious tracking
required.

What it does:
Every time you shift your weight, reach overhead, catch yourself mid-stumble, or roll across the ground, this system lights up.
It tells your brain:

- The angles of your joints
- The stretch of your muscles
- The pressure running through your limbs

With this data, your brain can predict, adjust, and refine movement in real time.

Why it matters:
Without proprioception, you would feel disconnected from your own body—as if moving through fog.
Balance would blur. Coordination would unravel. Movement would become guesswork.

But when you crawl, climb, balance, or vault across varied terrain, you sharpen this internal map—
You become faster, more stable, and more adaptive in unpredictable environments.

Proprioception isn't thinking about movement.
It's feeling movement—before thought ever arrives.

> **Mini-Integration: Balance Within**
>
> In the instant his foot slipped,
> his **vestibular system** screamed tilt and acceleration.
> His **proprioceptive system** mapped joint angles and shifting limb positions in real time.

But this wasn't just *awareness*.
It was *action*.

Within milliseconds:

- ✦ **Muscle spindles** sensed the sudden stretch.
- ✦ **Golgi tendon organs** registered the spike in tension.
- ✦ **Reflex arcs** fired through the spinal cord—sending movement instructions before the brain even got the memo.

He didn't decide to adjust.
He was already adjusting.

His shoulder tucked.
His center of mass rolled over the hip.
His foot swept wide and found the earth again.

This wasn't luck.
It wasn't instinct alone.

It was **layered intelligence**—built from years of crawling, balancing, climbing, falling, recovering.
It was the internal symphony of sensation and reflex saving him before he even knew he needed saving.

Balance isn't stillness.
Balance is dynamic, reflexive, and deeply felt—
a masterpiece of movement crafted faster than thought.

Modern Mismatch—The Cost of Sensory Deprivation

Your sensory systems evolved to interpret a rich, ever-changing environment—texture beneath your feet, shifting light, wind on skin, sounds echoing across distance.

But modern life often starves this system—or over-whelms it.

Flat floors. Constant noise. Predictable lighting. Headp-hones. Screens.
The result? Sensory undernourishment—or overload.

Natural movement in complex environments restores the balance. It feeds the senses with challenge, novelty, and information—the raw materials the brain needs to stay sharp, responsive, and alive.

Afferent and Efferent Signals: The Reflex Loop

- **Afferent nerves** carry incoming sensory signals **to the spinal cord**.

- **Efferent nerves** carry outgoing motor commands **from the spinal cord** back to muscles.

In a true reflex:

- Sensory input enters the spinal cord.

- Processing happens **at the spinal level**, not in the brain.

- Corrective motor action is sent back out almost instantly—within milliseconds.

The brain **only finds out afterward** what the body already did to survive.

Why This Matters

When the hiker slipped,
his muscles, tendons, and spinal circuits responded in perfect sync—long before conscious thought had a chance to intervene.

He didn't choose to tuck and roll.
His body knew.

Years of crawling, balancing, climbing, and falling had sculpted reflex patterns too fast for awareness,
too refined for panic.

This is the power of movement training—
not just strength,
but a symphony of instinct tuned through repetition.

Reflexes are your first line of defense.
You don't think your way out of danger.
You train your way into survival.

Reflexes—How the Body Reacts Before the Mind

In the split second after a slip, stumble, or sudden threat, your body doesn't wait for permission.

It moves before you know it.

This is the power of **reflex arcs**—ancient survival circuits hardwired into your spinal cord.
They bypass the brain, delivering action at the speed of life itself.

Muscle Spindles: The Stretch Sensors

Tiny sensors are embedded deep within your muscles.

Their job? Detect how much—and how fast—a muscle is stretching.

When that stretch happens too quickly—like when your foot slips—
they fire immediate signals to your spinal cord, triggering protective contraction.

They don't ask.
They act.

They say:
Stretch detected! Stabilize now—before damage sets in.

Golgi Tendon Organs: The Tension Sensors

Tucked where muscle meets tendon, these sensors monitor strain and force.

When tension surges toward a dangerous threshold,
they send a message:
Stop contracting. Let go. Protect the joint.

They are your built-in pressure valves—
ensuring that strength never turns into self-destruction.

Visual System: The Primary Scout

What it is:
The visual system includes your eyes, optic nerves, and the brain regions that process visual information.

What it does:
It gathers an immense amount of data in real time:
– Light, color, shape, and motion
– Distance, depth, speed, and direction
– Environmental threats and navigational options

But vision isn't passive.
It doesn't just *see* the world—it *interprets* and *predicts* it.

It tells you:
– Where obstacles are
– How fast they're moving
– Whether that leap is possible—or a mistake

Why it matters:
Even the most capable movers become vulnerable if they can't read their surroundings.
When your visual system is sharp, movement becomes proactive—not just reactive.

Training vision through dynamic environments—scanning, adjusting, recalibrating on the fly—
builds a brain that doesn't just *see* movement,
but anticipates it.

Vision isn't observation.
Vision is strategy in motion.

How Vision Builds Movement Intelligence
Vision is more than seeing—it's interpreting the world for action. To do this, your brain uses both biological hardware and real-time pattern recognition.

The Hardware: Anatomy of the Eye

Your eyes gather light through the cornea and lens, which focus images onto the retina—a thin layer at the back of the eye filled with photoreceptors:

- Rods detect light and motion in low light (mainly in the peripheral field).
- Cones detect color and fine detail (concentrated in the fovea, at the center of vision).

Signals from the retina travel via the optic nerve to the brain's visual centers—first the thalamus (for filtering), then the primary visual cortex, and onward to areas that assess movement, shape, depth, and threat.

The Software: Ecological Dynamics

Your brain doesn't just record images. It extracts *meaningful movement information* from the visual field—especially what matters for action.

Invariants

Stable visual properties that don't change even when your angle or speed changes.

Example: The shape of a rock remains the same whether you approach it quickly or slowly.

Affordances

Opportunities for action in the environment, based on both object properties and your capabilities.
Example: A branch "affords" gripping or vaulting only if it's within reach and strong enough to support your weight.

> **When you glance at a surface, you don't see** *just a surface*—**you know whether you can crawl across it, balance on it, or leap to it.**
> **That's affordance detection in action.**

Focal vs. Peripheral Vision

- Focal vision is narrow and detail-focused—used for planning and targeting (e.g., where to place a foot).

- Peripheral vision is wide-angle and motion-sensitive—used for orientation and detecting changes (e.g., something rushing at you from the side).

Effective movers switch rapidly between these modes— tracking threats, scanning landing zones, and sensing stability without needing to consciously "look."

Why This Matters

Your vision isn't just passive input.

It's a prediction engine, a movement guide, and a constant scanner for what matters now.

When you train in complex environments—navigating branches, vaulting walls, reacting to shifting terrain—you train your brain to see what matters for movement, not just what's in view.

Auditory System: The Silent Guide

What it is:
The auditory system processes sound through the ears and translates it into spatial and environmental awareness.

What it does:
In movement, sound isn't background noise. It's critical information:

– The *crack* of a breaking branch behind you
– The *rush* of moving water ahead
– The *grind* of shifting gravel underfoot

The auditory system helps you:
– Detect threats or opportunities beyond your field of vision
– Confirm—or contradict—what your eyes report
– Add speed, depth, and direction to your perception of space

Why it matters:
Hearing expands your awareness into the unseen.
Auditory cues stitch the world together faster than sight alone.

When you train in rich sensory environments—crawling across loose stone, navigating forest trails, reacting to natural echoes—
you're not just building physical agility.
You're wiring your brain for rapid, multi-dimensional spatial processing.

Movement without sound is incomplete.
The body doesn't just *see* the world—
it *listens* to it.

Mini-Integration: External Awareness

As the hiker fell,
his eyes caught the blur of the slope,
while his ears registered the crack of branches and the rush of displaced leaves.
The visual system predicted where the ground would rise to meet him.
The auditory system confirmed what lay beyond his line of sight.
Together, they allowed him not just to react—
but to *anticipate* his recovery.
He scanned. He adjusted. He rolled with the terrain—
before conscious calculation could even begin.

Navigation isn't just seeing.
Navigation is *sensing* a world too vast for one sense alone.

Tactile and Interoceptive Systems: Feeling the World Within and Without

How Your Brain Locates Sound in Space

Your ears don't just hear *sound*.
They detect *where* that sound is coming from—and how fast it's moving.

Here's how the auditory system builds a 3D sound map:

Interaural Time Difference (ITD)

Sound reaches one ear **slightly earlier** than the other.
Your brain measures the microsecond delay—sometimes

just 0.01 milliseconds—
to determine **horizontal direction** (left/right).

If a branch snaps to your right, your right ear hears it first.
The brain triangulates that difference.

Interaural Level Difference (ILD)

Sound is also **louder** in the ear it hits first.
Your skull blocks some of the sound from reaching the far ear, creating a volume difference.
This helps your brain refine the **angle and proximity** of the sound source.

The Pinna Effect

Your outer ear (pinna) subtly reshapes sound based on **vertical position.**
Was the rustle **above you** in the trees, or below near the ground? The unique folds of your ear filter sound differently depending on elevation, giving your brain vertical spatial clues.

Cortical Processing

All this data travels through the **auditory nerve** to the brainstem and up to the **auditory cortex.**
There, it's combined with visual and proprioceptive information
to create a seamless model of your environment.

Why This Matters
Sound isn't just background.
It's a directional *warning system*, a spatial *GPS*, and a guide to unseen danger or opportunity.

> When you move through the world—especially fast, especially blind—
> your ears help your brain build the map your eyes can't always see.

Tactile System: The Skin's Conversation

What it is:
The tactile system is built from receptors in your skin—specialized to detect touch, pressure, temperature, vibration, and texture.

What it does:
Every surface you touch—
the bark of a tree, the grit of stone, the softness of leaf litter—
sends messages to your brain about what you're contacting and how.
Tactile feedback tells you:

- Where your body meets the world
- How much pressure you're applying
- Whether friction is helping or betraying you

It refines grip, balance, and movement moment by moment—without thought.

Why it matters:
Without tactile feedback, your hands would slip, your feet would miss, and your connection to the environment would blur. Training through crawling, climbing, balancing barefoot, and carrying objects of varied shapes and textures fine-tunes this feedback loop.

Movement without tactile awareness is like playing piano with numb fingers.
Touch transforms intention into *precision*.

Interoceptive System: The Hidden Compass of Self

What it is:
The interoceptive system monitors your internal state—tracking signals from the heart, lungs, gut, blood vessels, and muscles.

It tells you:

- How fast your heart is beating
- How deep you're breathing
- Whether you're hungry, thirsty, overheating, exhausted, or in pain

What it does:
As you move, interoception helps calibrate your capacity:

- How hard you can push
- When you need to slow down
- Whether you're drifting toward danger—dehydration, overheating, or collapse

It links internal physiology to emotion,
and teaches you to *listen inwardly*—even while navigating the outer world.

Why it matters:
Interoception is the invisible foundation of endurance, regula-

tion, and resilience.
It doesn't shout. It *whispers*—but only if you've trained yourself to hear it.

Movement challenges that raise internal strain—long carries, uphill scrambles, crawling under resistance—don't just build toughness. They sharpen your sensitivity to your body's truth.

To master movement, you must first master yourself—starting with the signals your own body *whispers before it screams.*

Mini-Integration: Awareness Within

As the hiker fell,
it wasn't just the external world he sensed.

His hands prepared for impact, tension adjusting without command.
His feet searched midair for friction, angling toward a landing.
His heart thundered warnings of urgency.
His lungs pulled sharp, reflexive breaths to reset balance and breath.

Touch anchored him to the surface of the world.
Internal sensation anchored him to himself.

Together, they gave him the self-awareness to absorb shock, redirect momentum, and rise back into motion.

Movement is not just outward exploration.
Movement is the art of feeling the world—and yourself—at once.

Nociceptive System: Pain as a Guide, Not a Punishment

What it is:
The nociceptive system is your internal alarm system—
a network of specialized nerve fibers (nociceptors) that detect
tissue damage or its threat.

What it does:
When you strain, burn, cut, or absorb force—
nociceptors fire signals to your nervous system.
The result is pain—but pain isn't punishment. It's information.

Pain tells you:

- "You've gone too far."
- "Protect this area now."
- "Adapt your strategy before it breaks you."

Why it matters:
Without nociception, you wouldn't know to pull back.
You wouldn't learn from near-injury.
You wouldn't evolve wiser movement over time.

Effective natural movement practice—crawling, climbing,
balancing—trains you to move near your edge,
not past it.
To recognize when intensity must yield to intelligence.
To trust pain not as the enemy—
but as a teacher.

> Pain is not the failure of movement.
> Pain is the *mentor* that shapes survival into wisdom.

The Emotional Loop—Mood, Perception, and Movement

Movement doesn't happen in isolation. Your emotional state—stress, anxiety, joy, or calm—alters how you perceive the world and how your body responds to it. But the loop runs both ways.

Research in neurorehabilitation and trauma-informed movement shows that intentional movement can *change* emotion and perception. A slumped posture dulls your attention. A confident gait lifts your mood. A moment of stillness re-centers your breath—and your mind.

Every movement you make carries a signature of your internal state. And every deliberate action has the power to reshape that state.

Movement changes mood.
Mood changes perception.
Perception reshapes movement.
This is the triad of embodied intelligence.

Mini-Integration: Survival's Last Voice

As the hiker fell,
the risk of impact was real.
Nociceptors in his skin, joints, and muscles stood ready—
poised to sound the alarm if contact turned to damage.

But the strike never came.
His balance, his spatial awareness, his reflexes—refined by years of movement—redirected the danger just enough.

He didn't bypass pain through luck.
He did it through readiness.

Pain was there—not as a punishment,
but as a possibility.
A silent warning signal guiding every micro-adjustment
of his descent.

The nociceptive system stood vigilant—
the final sentinel in the chain of survival,
waiting to act if every other safeguard failed.

Pain is not the enemy of movement.
Pain is the compass that keeps movement honest.

The Sensory Symphony: Awareness Becomes Action

Movement does not begin with muscle.
Movement begins with awareness.

Before a foot lifts,
before a shoulder drops,
before a body bends into the arc of survival—
the orchestra of the senses is already playing.

The **vestibular system** feels gravity's tilt,
guiding posture before balance is even lost.

The **proprioceptive system** maps every joint and tendon in
space, locating self before the world can close in.

The **visual system** reads the terrain ahead,
catching the blur of earth and opportunity in a single glance.

The **auditory system** listens for what can't be seen,
hearing dangers that eyes might miss.

PHYSIOLOGY OF PURPOSE

The **tactile system** connects the body to the surface,
reading friction, pressure, texture—refining every adjustment.

The **interoceptive system** whispers from within,
monitoring breath, heartbeat, fatigue—the inner tides of life.

And the **nociceptive system** stands watch at the threshold,
ready to sound the alarm if survival falters.

In the moment of the hiker's fall,
all seven systems converged—
faster than thought,
more ancient than choice.

They mapped the world.
They mapped the self.
They mapped the way out—
rolling, adjusting, recovering—before the mind could catch up.

The brain didn't choose survival.
The senses **ensured** it.

> You are not a thinker who moves.
> You are a mover who feels the world first,
> solves the unknown second,
> and thinks about it only after the body has already
> lived it.

Movement is not the product of thought.
It is the force that shapes it.
A symphony too quick for words,
too beautiful for conscious control.

You are alive not because you think first—
but because you **move first**.
And in every movement,
your senses sing the ancient song that made life itself possible.

The Physiology of Purpose

Move like it matters.
Because inside you—it always does.

Movement makes the brain.
Movement refines the brain.
Movement preserves the brain.

Movement is awareness made real.
Awareness becomes action.
Action becomes survival.

Across every stage of life—
you don't just move through the world.
You move to become who you are.
And who you are
is built by how you move.

CHAPTER 4

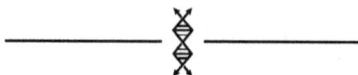

THE NERVOUS SYSTEM IN ACTION

He saw the wolves, and the decision to run wasn't a decision at all.

In a flash, the nervous system surged forward.
His pupils dilated, flooding his retinas with light.
The visual cortex sharpened contrast and depth perception, finding paths before the body even moved.
Cervical reflexes aligned his head and neck with the target of escape. Auditory centers filtered out background noise, tuning in to threats. The vestibular system stabilized his gaze mid-sprint, letting his eyes stay fixed eve n as his head bounced.

His heart pounded faster—nerves signaling the sinoatrial node to accelerate. Blood vessels constricted in the gut and skin, shunting blood to his limbs. His bronchioles opened. Breath deepened. Oxygen surged. Adrenal glands, wired by sympathetic nerves, dumped catecholamines into the bloodstream—epinephrine and norepinephrine, unlocking raw power.

Motor units fired with explosive synchrony.
Flexors and extensors alternated like pistons.
Reflex arcs shortened their thresholds.
Even his pain tolerance rose—nociceptive pathways muted, in case injury came second to survival.

The sprint wasn't just muscular.
It was neural.
Every step he took was a product of coordinated command—from the brainstem to the spine to the skin.
And it all began the moment his senses shouted the message:
Move. Now.

The Nervous System: The Body's Living Command Network

Movement, survival, adaptation—none of it happens without a system designed to sense, decide, and act.
The nervous system is that system.

It's not just a web of wires.
It's a living command network—dynamic, intelligent, and deeply embodied—reaching from brain to skin, from muscle to gut. It listens, it directs, it adjusts—every second you are alive.

When you sprint from danger, it triggers the surge.
When you crouch in silence, it sharpens your senses.
When you step forward after the threat has passed, it decides whether it's truly safe to heal.

Every signal, every shift, every adaptation—begins here.

To understand how the body moves through fear, through fatigue, through recovery,
we begin with its two great modes of command:

The Central Nervous System, the seat of interpretation and initiation
The Peripheral Nervous System, the messenger between the world and the will

Together, they form the command within.

Central Nervous System (CNS): The Command Center

The central nervous system is composed of the **brain and spinal cord**—the structural core of your mind and movement.

It does more than relay information.
It **integrates sensory input, generates motor output**, and **stores experience** as memory, strategy, and adaptation.

This is the seat of decision-making.
The place where raw sensation becomes meaning—
and meaning becomes movement.

It is not just the receiver.
It is the **interpreter**, the **strategist**, the **mind behind the motion.**

Peripheral Nervous System (PNS): The Messenger Network

The peripheral nervous system branches outward from the spinal cord, reaching every corner of the body.

It divides into two roles:
Sensory nerves bring information in.
Motor nerves carry commands out.

Some signals are voluntary.
Others bypass your awareness entirely.

The PNS doesn't make decisions—
It delivers them with speed and precision.

It's how the foot lifts.
How the hand grips.
How the lungs slow when the heart says, *"We're safe."*

Together, the CNS and PNS form a continuous loop:

- Sense the world (input)
- Decide what to do (integration)
- Act on the world (output)
- Receive new feedback (adjustment)

This loop fires thousands of times per second—
whether you're sprinting for your life
or strolling through a sunlit field.

Movement isn't separate from sensation.
Movement *is* sensation transformed into action.

Somatic Nervous System: Movement by Choice

What it is:
The somatic system governs voluntary movement.
Every deliberate action—
leaping over a fallen tree,
reaching for a handhold,
crouching to stay unseen—
originates here.

But it doesn't just send commands.
It also receives them:

- Proprioceptive signals from muscles and joints
- Touch from the skin
- Visual and auditory guidance

The somatic system is your conscious interface with the world.

Why it matters:
When you *choose* to move, the somatic system makes it real.
It lets you shape your environment.
It lets you respond with intelligence, grace, and precision.

Without it, you'd be trapped inside your body—
aware, but unable to act.

Movement practice refines this system—
tightening the bridge between thought and action
until they feel like one.

Somatic movement is the mind's signature—
written into the world through muscle, motion, and intent.

Sliding Filament Theory Meets Biotensegrity: How Movement Happens

When you choose to move, vaulting a log, sprinting across a rocky trail, or simply rising from the ground. Your nervous system sends the command.
But how does that command actually become motion?

It begins with a spark:
A motor neuron fires.
The signal travels down the nerve to the neuromuscular junction, where it releases acetylcholine.
That neurotransmitter crosses the tiny gap and binds to receptors on the sarcolemma (the muscle fiber's membrane).

In response, an electrical impulse races along the fiber, diving deep through T-tubules to reach the sarcoplasmic reticulum. There, calcium ions flood out unleashing the true engine of movement.

Actin and myosin filaments, the muscle's internal scaffolding, begin to slide past one another.
Each myosin head grabs, pulls, releases, and resets—ratcheting the fiber shorter and generating force.

This is the classic **Sliding Filament Theory**, the molecular choreography behind every contraction.

But there's more to the story.

The body is not a stack of levers. It's a dynamic, tension-integrated structure, a tensegrity system.
Muscles do not act alone. They transmit force through fascia, connective tissue, and bone, distributing tension across the entire body.

When you leap or land, when you adjust mid-crawl, you aren't isolating individual muscles, you're orchestrating a global shift in tension and compression:

- Tendons stretch and recoil.
- Fascia transmits force across distant chains.
- Joints stabilize not through brute strength, but through balanced tensional harmony.

Biotensegrity explains what levers cannot:
That movement is not generated by force acting *on* bones, but by a continuous conversation of tension *through* the system.

Sliding filaments create contraction. Biotensegrity distributes that force into integrated, adaptable motion.

Movement happens not from isolated muscle pull, but from the body's ability to balance tension, stabilize structure, and flow power through an ever-changing, responsive architecture.

Your nervous system sends the command. Your sliding filaments power the contraction.
Your tensegrity system transforms that contraction into movement through the world.

The Hierarchy of Wholeness

Humans like hierarchies.

We are taught:
The brain controls the body.

The nerves command the muscles.
The muscles move the bones.

But the living body is not so simple.

Every level—cell, tissue, muscle, fascia, bone, nerve,
speaks to every other.
No system works alone. No system sits "above" the rest.

The nervous system is not the master.
The fascia is not the servant.
The muscles are not mere motors.
The bones are not fixed levers.

Instead, the body behaves as an intelligent, adaptive
whole.

This is what biotensegrity means:
A living mesh of tension and compression spanning from
micro to macro, from cell to system.

A pull at one point echoes everywhere.
An adaptation in one area reshapes the whole.
Injury is systemic. Healing is systemic. Movement is
systemic.

This is why you cannot truly isolate strength, balance,
mobility, or awareness.
Every change, every adaptation, rises through the entire
network.

There is no master system.
There is only the beautiful intelligence of life woven
through your every breath, every step, every choice to
move.

How Muscles Contract—Key Terms

Motor Unit
A single motor neuron and all the muscle fibers it controls.

Sarcolemma
The membrane of a muscle fiber.

Actin & Myosin
The protein filaments responsible for muscle contraction.

Neuromuscular Junction
The connection point between a motor neuron and a muscle fiber. This is where nerve signals jump the gap and tell muscles to contract.

Acetylcholine (ACh)
A neurotransmitter is released at the neuromuscular junction. It binds to receptors on the muscle fiber's surface, triggering the contraction signal.

T-Tubules (Transverse Tubules)
Microscopic tunnels that carry the electrical signal deep into the muscle fiber, ensuring the whole cell responds at once.

Sarcoplasmic Reticulum (SR)
An internal reservoir inside muscle cells that stores calcium. When activated, it releases calcium to initiate contraction.

Calcium Ions (Ca^{2+})
The key that unlocks muscle contraction. When released from the SR, calcium binds to regulatory proteins on the

muscle filaments, allowing them to slide and generate force.

Sliding Filament Theory
The classic model of muscle contraction: myosin (thick filament) pulls actin (thin filament) inward, shortening the muscle. This "sliding" requires ATP and repeats millions of times in every movement.

Fascia
The connective tissue web that surrounds and links muscles, bones, and organs. In the biotensegrity model, fascia transmits and distributes force more than bones do.

Integrins
Proteins that anchor the inside of a cell to the outside matrix. They link the muscle's internal structure to fascia, allowing whole-body force transfer, not just local contraction.

Biotensegrity
A structural model where bones float in a web of tension (fascia and muscle), rather than acting as levers. Movement emerges from modulated tension, not rigid mechanical push-pull.

Narrative Prelude:

The sprint was over, the forest still, but the storm inside him raged on. His chest heaved, pulling air into burning lungs. His heart slammed against his ribs, pounding a rhythm for battle, not rest. His hands shook from primal effort, muscles primed for another wave of violence. But nothing came—only silence. In that silence, a question rose—not with words but sensation: Am I safe? Inside, command systems shifted without waiting for a mental answer. The sympathetic surge that had fueled his sprint began to soften. Slowly, cautiously, baroreceptors sensed the slowing blood rush, while mechanoreceptors whispered that perhaps the emergency had passed. In the brainstem, the pons and medulla recalibrated, urging slower inhalations and deeper exhalations, returning life's rhythm toward balance.

The vagus nerve, quiet during the sprint, stirred, testing its strength against lingering fear. Was it time to recover? Every breath was a negotiation. Every heartbeat raised questions. Still crouched among the trees, the hiker listened with every cell of his being. The nervous system was orchestrating survival in two directions: ready to sprint if a new threat appeared and to heal if safety proved real. This was no binary switch but a living dance—performed after every effort, danger, and moment where life decides between vigilance and restoration. Survival is not a moment, but a symphony, a command that never truly ends. In that symphony, the nervous system holds the baton, guiding the body, mind, and self across the line between fear and freedom.

They're the "ghostwriters" of fluid movement.

Autonomic Nervous System: Movement Beyond Choice

What it is:
The autonomic system regulates everything you don't consciously control—your heart rate, breathing patterns, blood

pressure, digestion, immune function, and more. It represents the body's deep intelligence—acting faster than thought and wiser than will.

The autonomic system has two major branches:

- Sympathetic Division ("Fight or Flight")
- Parasympathetic Division ("Rest and Recover")

What it does:
When danger appears—
when the wolves rise, when your foot hits the ground and your lungs gasp for air—
the sympathetic system takes command.

- Pupils dilate to widen your visual field
- Blood shunts from the digestive organs to the skeletal muscles
- Heart rate climbs, and breathing deepens
- Glucose is liberated from storage
- Reflexes sharpen

When the danger fades—
when your breath slows and your posture softens—
the parasympathetic system returns.

- Blood flows back to the gut
- The heart decelerates
- Muscles relax
- Repair begins
- Immunity recalibrates

Why it matters:
You don't get to choose these shifts.
But you *can* train them.

Through movement, breathwork, environmental stress, and conscious recovery,
you teach the autonomic system to move smoothly between extremes—how to mobilize when needed and how to restore when safe.

Autonomic resilience forms the basis of all other types of resilience.
It's what enables you to fight and heal.
It's why your body knows when to maintain tension—and when to finally release it.

> **Mini-Integration: Conscious and Unconscious Survival**
> As the hiker sprinted,
> he chose to run—*somatic control.*
> But his heart raced, his lungs flooded with air, his blood diverted from gut to muscle—all without permission—*autonomic control.*
>
> When he crouched and waited in the woods,
> he chose to slow his breath—*somatic control.*
> But his body negotiated internally whether it was truly safe to shift out of fight mode—*autonomic control.*
>
> Survival is not just thinking and moving.
> It is thinking, moving, and enduring inside a continuous negotiation between conscious choice and unconscious command.
> **Mastery comes not just from controlling the body—but from respecting and refining the systems that control you.**

Interneurons—Hidden Architects of Fast Movement

When you step on a sharp rock and recoil before you even feel pain—that's the work of interneurons.

These are the relay specialists of the spinal cord and brain, forming lightning-fast circuits between sensory input and motor output:

- **Spinal Reflexes**: Interneurons connect sensory receptors in the skin or muscle directly to motor neurons—allowing you to move without waiting for the brain.

- **Central Pattern Generators**: These spinal networks coordinate rhythmic actions like crawling, walking, or running.

- **Inhibitory Control**: Some interneurons *suppress* movement patterns, helping with balance, focus, and precision.

You don't feel them working—but they're always there: coordinating action, accelerating reaction, and protecting the system from delay.

Sympathetic Activation: Tactical Reorientation for Movement

When survival demands action,
the nervous system doesn't simply raise an alarm.

It reorients the entire physiology toward one singular purpose: movement with intent.

This isn't a partial change. It is a full-body shift—a temporary rewiring of the self for one mission: **survive.**

Hormonal Reorientation: Readiness for Battle

The moment danger triggers sympathetic activation:

- **Cortisol** floods circulation—not to damage, but to *prime* tissues for rapid, sustained output.

- **Glucagon** rises, mobilizing glucose stores to feed the muscles.

- **Insulin** is suppressed, allowing blood sugar to be available for performance, not storage.

This is not an energy system built for comfort.

This is fuel allocation under threat—

the same metabolic machinery from Chapter 1, now firing at full intensity.

Energetic Reorientation: Power Before Efficiency

Under sympathetic control:

- The **ATP-PC system** activates instantly, delivering explosive power.

- **Glycolysis** accelerates, flooding muscles with lactate, *not a waste product, but a fuel in motion.*

- The **Cori Cycle** activates, recycling lactate at the liver into glucose, ensuring backup reserves remain intact even in the middle of the sprint.

These systems don't compete.
They **stack and overlap**, creating an energetic storm—
primed to burn at any cost, if survival demands it.

Sensory Reorientation: Perception Sharpens
Under sympathetic dominance, the sensory world sharpens:

- **Vestibular system:** Heightened sensitivity to head position and acceleration—critical for sudden agility.

- **Visual system:** Pupils dilate, widening the field of view, increasing low-light vision, and motion detection.

- **Auditory system:** Filters background noise to prioritize sudden changes, like snaps, cracks, and shifts in the environment.

This is the **sensory orchestra of Chapter 3**—now re-tuned for urgency and threat.
Focus narrows.
Perception intensifies.
Reaction becomes the prime directive.

Cognitive Reorientation: Thought Narrows for Action

- **Prefrontal cortex** activity downshifts—long-term planning gives way to short-term execution.

- **Midbrain and brainstem circuits** accelerate reflexive responsiveness.

- Complex thinking gives way to direct action.

Your brain doesn't want debate.
It wants you moving—*now*.

Why This Matters

Sympathetic activation is not chaos.
It is *precision survival intelligence.*
The heart doesn't just beat harder—it redirects.
The eyes don't just see—they scan for threat.
Muscles don't just tense—they prepare to *launch.*

Even your mitochondria—your microscopic power plants—
shift behavior in response to this demand.
This isn't "stress."
This is *choreographed, adaptive stress*—designed to make
movement under pressure not just possible, but inevitable.

Parasympathetic Activation: The Dance Back to Restoration

But survival through action is only half the equation.
The body's brilliance lies not just in *escaping* danger—
but in knowing how to *recover* once the danger is gone.

The parasympathetic system does not shout.
It whispers.

When the world calms,
the body doesn't collapse.
It rebuilds.
It rebalances.
It restores.

The vagus nerve activates.
The heart rate slows.
Blood returns to the gut.
Breathing deepens.
Muscles soften.
Learning begins.

This is not a weakness.
This is resilience—at the cellular level.

The Vagus Nerve—Conductor of Calm

Hidden deep within your body, extending from the brainstem to the gut, the **vagus nerve** serves as the **primary pathway for parasympathetic activation**—and it is one of the most crucial regulators of recovery, emotion, and resilience.

It's not just a nerve.
It's a lifeline for *downshifting* your physiology.

What It Does:

- Slows the **heart rate**
- Deepens and regulates **breathing**
- Stimulates **digestion**
- Suppresses **inflammation**

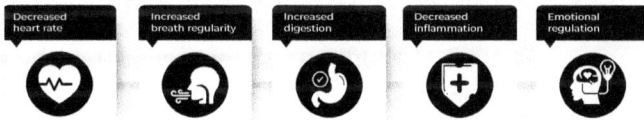

Links to **emotional regulation**, social connection, and even voice tone

When the vagus nerve is *active and responsive*, it signals safety. However, when it is **dysregulated**, the body struggles to shift out of the fight-or-flight response—even after the threat has passed.

Why It Matters for Movement:

Good vagal tone means faster recovery between sprints, rounds, or lifts

It means you can downshift from intensity into restoration, without getting stuck in sympathetic overdrive

It helps stabilize breathing, focus attention, and **regulate the nervous system on demand**

You don't just train your body.
You train your ability to return to calm.
And that training begins with listening to the **quiet power of the vagus nerve.**

Breath as the First Messenger

The shift begins with breath.

Mechanoreceptors in the lungs and chest sense the slower rise and fall of the chest.
Baroreceptors in the arteries detect the easing of blood pressure.
Together, they send a signal:

It might be safe now.

That signal rides the vagus nerve—the great parasympathetic highway—up toward the brainstem.
In the pons and medulla, the respiratory centers respond by

slowing the breath, deepening the rhythm, dialing down the alarm.

The body first listens to the breath and heartbeat.
If they whisper calmly, the rest will follow.

Breath isn't just air.
It's the body's first language for "You survived."

How the Brain Orchestrates Breath

Breathing isn't just about the lungs. It's brainstem intelligence in motion.

Your brainstem—specifically the pons and medulla oblongata— houses the control centers that generate and regulate your breathing rhythm.

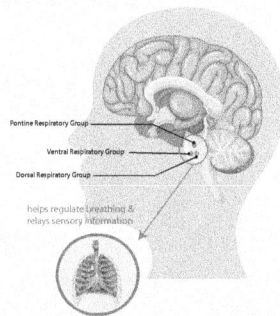

- ✦ **Pontine Respiratory Group (PRG): Located in the pons, this group fine-tunes breathing. It smooths transitions between inhalation and exhalation, adapting breathing patterns to emotional and environmental changes—whether you're resting, sprinting, or recovering after a close call.**

- ✦ **Dorsal Respiratory Group (DRG): Located in the medulla, this group regulates the rhythm for relaxed, involuntary breathing, particularly during rest and recovery.**

✦ **Ventral Respiratory Group (VRG): Also in the medulla, this center becomes active during forceful breathing, such as during sprints, effortful climbs, or high emotional stress.**

These centers adjust your breath before you're aware of the need, responding to CO_2 levels, blood pressure, muscle feedback, and even posture.

When breath changes, the brain listens.
And if the message is safety, the rest of the body follows.

The Spine: Neural Superhighway and Interoceptive Core

The spine is not just a structure.
It is sensation.
It is a signal.
It is the neural superhighway of survival and recovery.

Within the spinal column runs the spinal cord, connecting brain to body, body to brain.
Through its vertebral joints and fascia, thousands of mechanoreceptors feed constant updates into the nervous system.

Spinal motion = sensory input.
A dynamic spine sharpens proprioception, reorients balance, and tunes interoceptive awareness.

Breath and spinal motion are linked:
Each inhalation subtly extends the spine.
Each exhalation subtly releases it.

Movement here is not cosmetic—it is autonomic.
Free spinal motion influences:

- Vagal tone
- Breath rhythm
- Baroreceptor sensitivity
- Parasympathetic recovery

A locked spine locks the nervous system.
A mobile, responsive spine frees it.

This is why natural movement restores recovery:
Not just through rest, but through motion that speaks
to the spine, refining the conversation between breath,
balance, and the autonomic core.

When the spine moves well, the whole system listens.

Hormonal Rebalancing: From Readiness to Recovery

As parasympathetic activity deepens:

- **Cortisol levels drop**, signaling the end of emergency mode.
- **Insulin sensitivity returns**, allowing nutrients to flow into muscle cells for repair.
- **Growth hormone levels rise**, quietly activating recovery and regeneration.

The hormonal symphony that once primed the body for
movement now reshapes it through restoration—
not with urgency, but with precision and care.

Energy Reallocation: Repair Over Reaction

In sympathetic mode, energy is spent like a match—burn fast, burn now, survive at all costs.

In parasympathetic restoration, energy is budgeted with purpose:

- **Cellular repair takes priority.**
- **Mitochondrial biogenesis**—the creation of new energy factories—ramps up.
- **Glycogen stores** begin to refill, preparing muscles for future demands.
- The **lactate shuttle** still hums, but now it's not about fueling escape— it's about powering recovery.

Rest is not the absence of effort.
Rest is the redirection of energy toward resilience.

Sensory Integration: Rebuilding the World Map

With the threat gone, the senses begin their return from war:

- **Vestibular recalibration** restores postural balance and spatial ease.
- **Visual and auditory fields** expand, reintroducing peripheral awareness.
- **Interoceptive signals**—heart rate, breathing rhythm, internal tension—settle back into baseline.

- **Nociceptive pathways** transition from suppressing pain to monitoring for tissue repair and guiding recovery.

What was once a tunnel of survival
widens into a full-spectrum map of the world.

The nervous system doesn't just *survive* a threat—
it *rebuilds* its understanding of reality after the storm has passed.

Mini-Integration: The Two Halves of Mastery

True resilience demands both systems.

The sprint alone is not mastery.
The roll and recovery are not enough.
Without the return to calm, survival never becomes growth.

The nervous system must do more than fight for life—
it must *heal* for life to continue.

Strength is the sprint.
Wisdom is the recovery.
Movement is the dance between the two.

The Living Loop: Survival, Recovery, and Mastery

Movement is not a one-way street.
It is a living, breathing cycle:

You move to survive.
You survive to recover.

PHYSIOLOGY OF PURPOSE

You recover to adapt.
You adapt to move better.

The nervous system conducts every phase of this cycle—
guiding your body, your mind, and your awareness across the
invisible bridge from crisis to growth.

When the hiker sprinted for his life,
he unleashed every resource his body had ever built.
His sympathetic system sharpened his vision, accelerated his
heartbeat, primed his reflexes, and ignited his energy systems.
It didn't ask.
It didn't wait.
It acted.

And when the sprint ended,
what followed wasn't a collapse.
It was the careful, deliberate reorganization of life:

Breath slowing.
Heart rate recalibrating.
Blood flow returning to healing.
Sensory fields expanding once again.

The parasympathetic system took the baton, transforming
survival into restoration, and restoration into future resilience.

You are not just a body that moves.
You are a system that survives, restores, and evolves—
a living loop of action, awareness, and adaptation.

And every time you sprint, recover, breathe, and rebuild,
you refine that loop.
You train it to respond with greater strength, more profound
wisdom, and more freedom.

The nervous system doesn't just carry you through danger. It transforms danger into growth.

That is the true miracle of movement.

From Signal to Strength: How Neural Intent Becomes Motion

Every movement begins with a spark, an electrical impulse racing down a motor neuron.

But how does that signal become motion?

How does a decision to leap... become the leap?

It begins at the **neuromuscular junction, a microscopic** gateway where nerve meets muscle. When an action potential reaches the end of a motor neuron, it releases **acetylcholine** into the synaptic cleft. This neurotransmitter binds to receptors on the muscle fiber's membrane, triggering an electrical cascade across its surface.

That signal dives inward through **T-tubules**, reaching deep into the fiber's interior, where it activates calcium channels in the **sarcoplasmic reticulum**. Calcium floods the cell.

And with that flood, the machinery of motion unlocks.

Sliding Filament Theory describes what happens next:

- Calcium binds to troponin, exposing binding sites on actin filaments.
- Myosin heads, powered by ATP, latch on, pulling actin, a protein filament, inward like oars on a boat.
- Each pull is a contraction. Each release is a reset.

Millions of these interactions occur in synchrony across fibers, bundles, and fascial lines, creating not a single lever pull but a full-body orchestration of force.

But this is not a system of pulleys and hinges.

It is not a biomechanical machine of rigid levers and torque arms.

It is something far more adaptive.

It is **tensegrity** in motion.

More Than ACh—Other Neurotransmitters That Influence Movement

Content:
Acetylcholine is the prime mover of voluntary muscle contraction—but it's not the only neurotransmitter that shapes how we move, adapt, and perform.

- **Dopamine:** Fine-tunes movement precision and motivation. Deficits are central in Parkinson's disease.

- **Norepinephrine:** Heightens arousal, vigilance, and movement readiness—critical during sympathetic activation.

- **Serotonin:** Modulates pain perception, fatigue, and motor coordination.

- **Glutamate:** The brain's primary excitatory neurotransmitter—activates neurons throughout motor circuits.

✦ **GABA:** The main inhibitory neurotransmitter—helps prevent overactivation and tremors.

Together, these neurotransmitters form the chemical symphony that coordinates, refines, and stabilizes movement—moment by moment, motion by motion.

Biotensegrity: The Architecture of Adaptable Strength

In the traditional model, muscles pull on bones like ropes pulling levers. In the **biotensegrity model**, bones are not levers—they are floating struts within a web of continuous tension.

Fascia, not bone, transmits most of the force.
Tension, not compression, holds the system together.

Muscle contraction in this model is not just about pulling tendons in straight lines. It's about generating tension across a dynamic network that modulates stiffness, elasticity, and load distribution in real-time.

Even at the cellular level, **integrin proteins** connect the cytoskeleton of a muscle fiber to the surrounding extracellular matrix, allowing contraction to ripple across layers of fascia and distribute force throughout the tissue, joint, and limb.

Neural signals don't just activate a muscle.

They **tune the system,** adjusting global tension, joint stiffness, and structural responsiveness according to demand.

When you leap, you don't just push off the ground.

You release stored elastic energy from fascia, modulate pre-tension across chains, and allow recoil to assist propulsion.

This is not a machine.

This is **a living tensegrity field**, reshaped moment by moment by the nervous system.

Why This Matters

Understanding muscle contraction through this lens changes everything:

- It explains how movement remains efficient across angles, loads, and terrains.
- It reveals why joint health depends on **tensional balance**, not isolated strength.
- It shows that training isn't just about force production; it's about **tension modulation**, **tissue timing**, and **nervous system precision**.

Your nervous system doesn't just fire a signal to contract a muscle.

It composes a full-body solution to a movement problem, balancing fluidity, force, and feedback across a dynamic, intelligent structure.

From a single axon firing...

To a leap across unstable ground...

This is **neurobiotensegrity** in action.

The Physiology of Purpose

Move like it matters.
Because inside you, it always does.

Movement made the brain.
Movement refines the brain.
Movement preserves the brain.

Movement is awareness made real.
Awareness becomes action.
Action becomes survival.

Survival leads to recovery.
Recovery leads to adaptation.
Adaptation leads to freedom.

Across every stage of life—
you move to become who you are meant to be.

CHAPTER 5

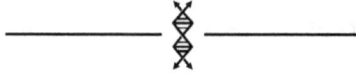

THE PROBLEMS THE WORLD POSES

The forest never stays still.
The terrain shifts beneath every step—
roots twist up from the earth,
stones slide in the mud,
branches arch across the path like silent, swinging gates.
No two steps are the same.
No two moments are the same.
Movement here isn't repetition.
It's problem-solving at the speed of life.

The hiker slows, not from fatigue,
but because the world demands more than speed.
It demands adaptability.

Ahead, a fallen tree blocks the trail.
A thick trunk. Rough bark.
Just high enough to make a clean step-over impossible.

No time to think, only feel.
Shift weight.

Adjust stride.

Vault—hands grazing bark, legs curling forward.

Land in a crouch.
One foot slips slightly on damp soil,
but the body adjusts midair.

No one taught him this sequence.
No coach diagrammed it.
No textbook outlined how to handle this tree, on this trail, on
this morning.

Movement is not a catalog of memorized patterns.
It is the ability to solve what the world demands in real-time.

This is what every actual mover trains for.
Not perfection.
Not performance.
Capability.

The ability to meet the unknown and move through it with
grace, strength, and intelligence.

Later, a wide stream interrupts the trail.
No bridge.

No easy crossing.

Rocks protrude above the rushing water—
slippery, uneven, irregularly spaced.

The hiker reads the stream the way a hunter reads tracks.
He maps the stones.

Visualizes the sequence: left foot, right foot, soft landing, slight pivot.

Then he moves.
Light. Fast. Committed.

Each step adjusts midair.
Each landing adapts to the real, not the planned, conditions.

Not every landing is perfect.
But every movement flows forward.

Because in the real world, perfect isn't the goal.
Adaptation is.

This is a capability:
The ability to move—
not because the world is easy,
but because you are adaptable.

The environment sets the problems.
If the body is trained,
it creates the solutions.

Movement—real movement—is not born from control.
It is born from the dance between pressure and possibility.

Affordances: How the World Offers You Movement

The body doesn't just move.
The body perceives *possibilities* for movement.

This truth runs deeper than any exercise program,
deeper than any coaching cue:

You don't move *through* the world.
You move *with* it.

In ecological psychology, these possibilities are referred to as
affordances.

An affordance is not the object itself—
it's the opportunity the object offers,
relative to your body, your skill, and your intent.

A low branch might afford a swing.
Or a duck-under.

A rock might afford a jump.
A vault.
A step.
A moment to rest.

A slope might afford a sprint.
Or a slide.

What you perceive—
and what you attempt—
depends on *who you are* in that moment:

- Your structure (height, limb length, joint mobility, body proportions)
- Your strength (how much force you can produce and absorb)
- Your coordination (timing, sequencing, spatial accuracy)
- Your emotional state (fear, confidence, presence)
- Your movement history (what your brain-body recognizes as possible)

Affordances are invitations, not commands.
The environment asks.
The body decides.

No two people see the same stream the same way.
No two people perceive the same wall as equally climbable.

Because movement isn't just about the environment.
It's about a *relationship*—
between your body
and the world it meets.

Perception–Action Coupling: Movement is Born From Meaning

When you move, you're not solving physics equations in your mind.
You're *feeling* affordances in real time:

Can I reach that ledge?
Can I land safely if I leap?
Will my foot hold If I push here?

These questions rarely rise to conscious thought.
They're embedded in perception itself.

Your brain doesn't just receive information—it extracts *meaning* from what you see, hear, and feel.
And that meaning transforms into movement
at breathtaking speed—faster than words can form.

This is **perception–action coupling**:

- Seeing opportunity
- Feeling possibility

- Moving into action without hesitation

Capability Is Not Strength Alone

Muscles matter.
Strength matters.
Skill matters.

But true capability is not just muscle or strength.
It's the ability to perceive and solve movement problems *at speed*.

A heavy deadlift means little
if you can't adjust midair while crossing a rocky stream.

A perfect squat means little
if you can't shift, pivot, and recover when a branch snaps underfoot.

Real-world movement is not a contest of repetition. It is a *conversation* between you and a changing world—and it's a conversation you must remain fluent in for life.

Mini-Integration: The Hiker's World

When the hiker sees the fallen tree,
he doesn't see a "problem" to brute-force through.
He sees an *affordance*.

Height.
Texture.
Angle.
All of it offers information.

His body reads the world
the way a musician reads a melody.

Movement doesn't emerge from force—
it emerges from a *relationship*.

Later, when he crosses the slick stones,
it's not maximal strength that saves him.
It's perception.
Recalibration.
A constant, fluid dialogue with the environment.

Every adjustment is a conversation
between the nervous system and the Earth.

This is not randomness.
This is *mastery* at work.

Capability is not the elimination of chaos.
Capability is moving skillfully *through* chaos.

Real-World Training: Building Capability Instead of Repetition

Strength without adaptability is brittle.
Skill without perception is hollow.

Real-world movement demands more than mechanical execution.
It demands **capability**—
the ability to perceive, adjust, and solve real problems under real-world pressure.

And that changes how you must train.

Traditional Exercise: Mastery Without Meaning

In most gyms, movement is divorced from environment:

Squats occur under fixed loads on flat, predictable surfaces.
Pull-ups are performed on symmetrical bars with uniform grips.
Lunges take place on even floors at consistent tempos under uniform conditions.

There's nothing wrong with building strength, coordination, or endurance in structured settings.
These are real adaptations.

But the world outside the gym doesn't behave like the world inside it.

The real world throws:

- Irregular surfaces
- Unpredictable obstacles
- Uneven friction
- Unexpected timing

The muscles trained in clean, rehearsed repetition do *not* automatically transfer to a chaotic reality.

Because what the world demands
is not just force production—
but rapid recalibration under uncertainty.

You can build a strong squat indoors.
But strength alone won't teach you how to land
when the ground gives way beneath your foot.

Capability is not a static output.
Capability is a living input—
reading, adjusting, solving
as the environment shifts.

Natural Movement: Reawakening Perception and Adaptation

Natural movement reconnects training to the world itself.
It forces you to:

- Scan surfaces dynamically
- Feel the weight and texture of real objects
- Adjust mid-movement to friction, slope, and feedback
- Solve problems you didn't plan for

This isn't randomness.
it's *pattern recognition under uncertainty*.

The nervous system sharpens.
The senses deepen.
The joints grow fluent in multi-planar stability.

The mind and body stop expecting symmetry and control—
and start expecting challenge, creativity, and solutions.

Training for Capability Means Training for Reality

If you want to move like it matters:

- Don't just squat on stable ground—squat where the earth gives a little
- Don't just pull from symmetrical bars—lift, drag, and carry uneven objects
- Don't just lunge at fixed tempos—crawl, jump, and respond to what your body feels

Training becomes a *conversation*, not a script.

And when you can adapt under pressure —
when your movements remain fluid as the world shifts —
you're no longer just fit.

You're capable.
And capability is what life demands.

Capability: Movement's True Purpose

The forest doesn't hand out repetitions.
It doesn't offer perfect conditions.
It offers you *problems*:

- A fallen tree to vault

- A crumbling slope to traverse

- A stream to cross, one shifting stone at a time

- A branch to catch—or duck under at the last second

Each step forward isn't a performance of memorized skills.
It's a conversation:

What does the environment offer?
What does my body perceive?
What solution can I create?

This is movement as it was meant to be:
Perception.
Decision.
Action.
Alive in real time.

In this world:

- Strength matters

- Coordination matters

- Endurance matters

But above all, **adaptability matters**.

The ability to read the world
and move *with* it—not against it—
is the birth of true capability.

Capability is not a perfect form.
Capability is fluent movement
through *imperfect* worlds.

Training that honors this truth doesn't just build muscles.
It builds minds.
It builds reflexes.
It builds bodies that *solve*, not just perform.

It creates movers, not lifters.
Explorers, not exercisers.
Humans who meet the unknown
with grace, power, and creativity.

What Is Ecological Dynamics?

Movement isn't just what you do to the world.
It's what you perceive and create with it.

This is the heart of a powerful idea in movement science:
Ecological Dynamics.

Ecological Dynamics merges:

- **Ecology—the relationship between an organism and its environment**
- **Dynamics—how systems change over time**

It teaches us:

Your movement doesn't originate from a fixed list of "skills" stored in your brain. It arises from the ongoing interaction between your body's capabilities and the environment's opportunities.

You don't "repeat" movement.
You solve movement.

Each step, each jump, each vault represents a new negotiation between the world, your body, and your intention.

Movement is not a blueprint.
Movement is a living conversation.

Training in real-world conditions—irregular, unpredictable, and varied—
doesn't just make you stronger.

It makes you more adaptive.
More perceptive.
More free.

This is the real path to capability.

The Physiology of Purpose

Move like it matters.
Because inside you, it always does.

Movement made the brain.
Movement refines the brain.
Movement preserves the brain.

Movement is awareness made real.
Awareness becomes action.
Action becomes survival.

Survival gives rise to recovery.
Recovery gives rise to adaptation.
Adaptation gives rise to freedom.

Freedom is the ability to meet the world—
not as you wish it were,
but as it is—
and move through it beautifully.

Across every stage of life,
you move to become who you are meant to be.

CHAPTER 6

———— ⚕ ————

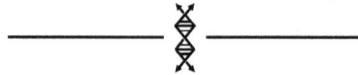

THE FITNESS ILLUSION

Two training sessions.
Two very different worlds.

Inside the gym, a man stands under bright lights, chalking his hands.
Today is "Arm Day."

- Dumbbell curls: strict form, fixed range, no surprises
- Cable pushdowns: elbows pinned, eyes locked straight ahead
- Concentration curls: heavy breathing, forehead veins pulsing

He grunts.
He strains.
He checks the mirror.

He finishes the set and flexes—first casually,
then a little more intentionally as another member walks by.

144

This is training for appearance:
muscle size, symmetry, and definition.
The body is a sculpture to be admired.

Just outside, in the park next door, another figure moves
differently.
Barefoot.
Eyes scanning the uneven ground.
Hands brushing a low branch for balance.

There's no mirror here.
No fixed repetitions.

Today's session includes:

- Crawling up a steep incline, adjusting hand and foot placement as rocks shift
- Vaulting over downed logs of unpredictable height and texture
- Lifting and carrying a dirt-slicked stone across uneven terrain
- Balancing across a narrow fallen tree, muscles twitching to stabilize

This body doesn't move for symmetry.
It moves for survival.
For adaptation.
For capability.

No two steps are identical.
No two landings are guaranteed.

Strength here isn't aesthetic.
It's functional.
It's relational.

From a distance, both bodies look "fit."
Both sweat.
Both strain.
Both work.

But the purpose underneath them is entirely different.

One trains to control one's appearance.
The other trains to meet the unknown.

Fitness, in the traditional sense, isn't wrong.
It's just incomplete.

Because life will never ask how much you can curl.
It will ask if you can adapt—if you can move, respond, and survive
when the ground shifts beneath you.

And for that, you need a body that can think, feel, and solve through movement.

Not just lift.
Not just sweat.
Solve.

Bodybuilding: Sculpted Strength vs. Adaptive Strength

When most people think of "fitness," they picture bodybuilding.

Big arms.
Broad shoulders.
Deep cuts between muscle groups.
A body that *looks* powerful, even statuesque.

And there's no question:

- Discipline is required
- Dedication is immense
- Hypertrophy is real and significant

Training for size demands:

- Consistent overload
- Structured nutrition
- Relentless attention to progression

It's a craft.
And it deserves respect.

But size is not equivalent to capability.
Because the world doesn't measure your symmetry.
It measures your ability to adapt.

What Bodybuilding Builds Well

- **Tissue Density –** Increased cross-sectional muscle mass
- **Glycolytic Efficiency –** Tolerance for moderate-intensity fatigue
- **Mental Discipline –** Routine mastery and consistency over time

Where Bodybuilding Falls Short

- **Rigidity over Fluidity** – Movements trained in isolation, not integration
- **Surface—Level Strength** – Force in fixed positions, but poor dynamic stability
- **Environmental Illiteracy** – No exposure to chaos, unpredictability, or terrain
- **Cost of Specialization** – Joint variability and connective elasticity are often sacrificed for size

The result?

An impressive machine—
on flat, controlled ground.

But a vulnerable mover—
when life introduces complexity:

- Uneven terrain
- Asymmetrical loads
- Split—second adjustments

The body you build reflects the world you prepare it for.
And traditional bodybuilding prepares you for a world of mirrors,
not mountains.

Natural Movement Response: Strength Beyond Aesthetics

Natural movement doesn't discard strength.
It builds strength where the *world* demands it—
across shifting loads, unstable surfaces, and unpredictable tensions.

Instead of isolating muscles for size alone,
natural movement integrates strength, stability, and adaptability into a unified system.

Key Natural Movements That Parallel and Often Surpass Bodybuilding Outcomes:

Lapping and Carrying Heavy Objects (e.g., river stones, fallen logs)

- Builds full-body strength through irregular, asymmetrical loading
- Trains grip, core, legs, and spine as a *coordinated unit* under shifting tension

Uneven Overhead Presses (e.g., lifting awkward branches or sandbags)

- Strengthens shoulders and stabilizers under dynamic, real-world loading
- Challenges anti-rotation and postural control during unstable lift paths

Loaded Crawling (e.g., with a weighted pack uphill)

- Develops shoulder girdle endurance and multiplanar trunk resilience
- Trains core-to-limb integration in low, adaptive positions

Ground-to-Overhead Lifts with Asymmetrical Objects (e.g., sandbags, natural stones)

- Conditions the body to respond to imperfect mass distribution
- Improves lift capacity and stability beyond linear barbell patterns

Why It Matters

- *Hypertrophy still happens*—but as a byproduct of building movement capacity, not chasing symmetry.
- *Joint variability is preserved*, reducing the overuse injuries common in fixed-pattern strength training.
- *Strength becomes elastic*—useful across multiple planes, positions, and unpredictable conditions.

You don't just get bigger.
You get better at being human.

The world will never test your biceps in isolation.
It will test your ability to stabilize, adapt, and move through inhospitable environments.

Natural movement trains you for the world, not the mirror.

Summary: Yes, Natural Movement Builds Muscle

While natural movement is celebrated for enhancing coordination, brain health, and adaptability, let's dispel a lingering myth: that it *can't* build muscle.

In truth, the *physiological environment* it creates may rival traditional hypertrophy training.

For decades, lactate was blamed for fatigue and soreness. But research now shows that lactate is not just recyclable fuel—
it may also be a messenger.

When you push into metabolic stress—
through high-volume crawling, loaded carries, and climbing efforts—
you're doing more than just tiring out. You're triggering adaptation.

This environment of lactate accumulation, cellular acidity, and hypoxic stress:

- **Stimulates growth hormone release**
- **Recruits Type II fibers, your most powerful, hypertrophy-prone units**
- **Promotes cell swelling, a key mechanical trigger for muscle growth**
- **May even activate gene expression via *lactylation*—an epigenetic signal for adaptation**

Lactate doesn't build muscle directly.
But it shows up when the conditions for growth are present—
and may help amplify those very conditions.

> Whether you're sprinting from wolves or hauling logs in silence,
> metabolic stress isn't something to avoid.
>
> It's a signal.
> A call to grow.
> A message:
> Adapt.

Powerlifting: Maximal Strength vs. Real-World Strength

If bodybuilding is the art of muscle display, powerlifting is the art of *maximal force*.

Three lifts rule this domain:

- **Squat**
- **Bench Press**
- **Deadlift**

Heavy.
Technical.
Relentless.

Powerlifters forge strength through *single-plane dominance*: vertical force production against unyielding, symmetrical loads.

And when it comes to demonstrating pure, absolute strength, few systems rival it.

- Bone density rises
- Connective tissues thicken
- Neuromuscular drive amplifies

It is brutal.
It is elegant.
And it deserves respect.

But life doesn't hand you a barbell.
It throws you asymmetry, instability, and chaos.
And this is where *maximal strength* meets its edge.

What Powerlifting Builds Well

- **Neuromuscular Efficiency** – Maximal fiber recruitment for peak effort
- **Tissue Reinforcement** – Strengthened ligaments and tendons under linear stress
- **Psychological Tenacity** – The mental toughness to grind through focused, high-stakes goals

Where Powerlifting Falls Short

- **Specificity Over Flexibility** – Mastery in fixed planes, dysfunction in dynamic settings
- **Reduced Movement Variability** – Repetitive patterns stiffen the body and limit adaptive options
- **Mass vs. Mobility Tradeoff** – Leverage often comes at the cost of agility and quick response

- **Energetic Rigidity** – Explosive strength lacks staying power in prolonged or creative demands

The result?

A *fortress* on the platform—
stable, powerful, unmoving.

But a *vulnerable system*
when the world becomes unpredictable:

- Scrambling up uneven terrain
- Reacting to a sudden fall
- Managing loads that shift, swing, or slip

Maximal strength is truly impressive.
But adaptive strength—strength that thinks, feels, and adjusts—is what life requires.

Natural Movement Response: Resilient Strength Beyond the Platform

Natural movement does not dismiss the value of maximal strength.
It develops **maximal *usable*** strength across unstable terrain, asymmetrical forces, and shifting body positions.

Instead of relying on stable platforms and predictable loads, natural movement trains the body to generate and stabilize force in *real-world chaos*.

Myofascial Continuity—Why the Body Moves in Chains

The body is not built in parts.
It is built in chains.

Every muscle fiber connects to fascia.
Fascia connects to bone, tendon, ligament, and back again.
No movement is isolated.

When you vault, sprint, or climb, it is never just "quads" or "glutes" or "shoulders" working.
It is whole-body coordination rippling across connected myofascial chains.

In sports science, this is often called **kinetic chains**:
Lines of tension and force that travel across regions of the body.

But this is more than mechanics.
It is a reflection of the body's true design:

Myofascial continuity, an unbroken web of connective tissue that integrates sensation, coordination, force, and resilience.

This is why:

- You cannot fully train balance on machines.
- You cannot fully train fluid strength on isolated lifts.
- You cannot transfer fixed gym movements into adaptive real-world capability.

Natural Movement trains these chains because it demands whole-body solutions to real-world problems.

When you crawl, vault, climb, and carry, you are not training muscles.
You are training myofascial intelligence, teaching your body to move as one.

Integration is what builds capability.
Isolation is what limits it.

Key Natural Movements That Parallel and Often Surpass Powerlifting Outcomes:

Heavy Object Lapping & Standing Lifts
(e.g., lifting a river boulder to chest height, adjusting stance to stabilize)

- Develops explosive hip, leg, and core strength
- Demands constant recalibration based on mass distribution and surface friction
- Trains *dynamic posture*, not static form

Asymmetrical Carries
(e.g., hauling a log on one shoulder across uneven terrain)

- Builds brutal core resilience and anti-rotational control
- Reinforces adaptive foot and ankle mechanics under unstable loads

Low-Gait Locomotion Under Load
(e.g., crawling with a weighted pack, duck-walking a heavy object)

- Trains hip strength, joint coordination, and multiplanar neuromuscular control

- Conditions the nervous system to organize effort across complex chains of movement

Dynamic Deadlifting Variations
(e.g., *sandbag pulls, odd-object ground-to-shoulder lifts*)

- Strengthens the posterior chain under inconsistent load paths
- Prepares the body for the unpredictable vectors of real-world tasks

Why It Matters

- *Maximal strength becomes adaptable*, not locked into a single lift or linear plane
- *Joint health improves* via variability, not compromised by over-repetition
- *Injury resilience skyrockets*—because the body trains for chaos, not just control

In the real world, the ground shifts.
The load shifts.
And your body must shift with it.

Natural movement doesn't just ask:
Can you lift heavy?

It asks:
Can you lift heavy, adjust mid-lift, stay stable when your footing slips, and solve under pressure?

That's not just strength.
That's resilient strength.
And it's the kind that *endures*.

The 600lb Squat vs. the Elbow Roll-Up

In 2022, I attended a seminar titled "Principles of Loaded Strength Training."
The entire weekend focused on three lifts:
the Deadlift, the Back Squat, and the Bench Press.

As part of the warm-up, one of the lead instructors introduced a preparatory drill:
The elbow roll-up.

Lying flat on your back, the task was to roll and prop yourself up onto one elbow—no momentum, no hands.
It was designed to activate the core and stabilize the shoulder before loading.

He called it the "first part of the Turkish Get-Up—just without the kettlebell."

And he couldn't do it.

He grunted, adjusted, and tried again.
Then laughed and said:
"This is harder than it looks."

When it was my turn, I performed it with ease.
He turned to the group and said:
"That's what it's supposed to look like."

I wasn't stronger than he was.
But I was more connected.
More coordinated.
More practiced.

That moment stayed with me.
Because strength isn't just what you can lift—

it's what you can *do* with your body,
starting from the ground up.

And the irony?
The movement they were struggling to name—the "elbow
roll-up"—is something I knew simply as the Get-Up.
It's a fundamental part of **Natural Movement**.

They didn't recognize it as that.
They didn't call it that.
But it's been here all along.

This is the more profound truth:
Natural movement is not a new invention.
It's a human inheritance.

But when we isolate strength into silos—into dogmatic
systems of output and metrics—
we forget the basics.
We overlook the movements that connect everything.

What MovNat did wasn't invent natural movement.
It *remembered* it.
And built a system around what was already ours.

Olympic Weightlifting: Power and Precision vs. Adaptability

If powerlifting is raw strength,
Olympic weightlifting is explosive precision.

Every rep demands:

- Absolute timing
- Maximal ground force production

- A flawless bar path
- Split-second decision-making under heavy loads

There's a kind of poetry to it:

- The clean pull from the floor
- The violent extension through the hips
- The effortless-seeming snap under the bar
- The stable catch overhead

Olympic lifters are, without question,
among the most powerful athletes on Earth.

But Olympic lifting occurs in a tightly controlled environment:

- Same barbell
- Same load geometry
- Same platform
- Same movement demands

The sport refines movement through extreme specificity.
While that specificity fosters brilliance,
it often restricts adaptability outside of its limited scope.

What Olympic Weightlifting Builds Well

- **Explosive Strength** – Rapid fiber recruitment for maximal power
- **Inter-Muscular Coordination** – Full-body synergy in complex kinetic sequences
- **Reactive Balance** – Stabilization under high-speed, high-load conditions

Where Olympic Weightlifting Falls Short

- **Controlled Environment Bias** – Always flat platforms, balanced loads, predictable surfaces
- **Narrow Adaptability** – Skills become hyper-specialized to barbell sequencing, not environmental randomness
- **Real-World Fragility** – Precision doesn't translate easily to shifting terrain, unstable loads, or unpredictable vectors
- **Mobility Tradeoffs** – Exceptional lift-specific mobility, but reduced freedom in multi-planar, real-world patterns

The result?

Explosive capability that dazzles—
but only when the rules are known.

- Uneven ground
- Asymmetrical loads
- Shifting friction
- Split-second environmental changes

These aren't just *different* conditions.
They speak a *different language*.

Olympic lifting builds a refined movement vocabulary. However, when the language of the world changes, the vocabulary can become brittle.

A perfect lift requires an ideal setup.
But the world rarely offers perfect setups.

Natural Movement Response: Explosiveness That Adapts

Natural movement doesn't reject power and precision.
It *evolves* them into a power that adapts in real time,
across unstable, shifting, and asymmetrical environments.

Instead of requiring a perfect platform and a predictable bar path,
natural movement trains the body to generate, redirect, and stabilize force
amid *dynamic, chaotic* conditions.

Key Natural Movements That Parallel and Surpass Olympic Weightlifting Outcomes:

Sprint Vaulting & Power Traverses
(e.g., running and vaulting over a fallen tree mid-stride)

- Builds explosive triple extension (hips, knees, ankles)
- Requires mid-flight adjustments based on height, angle, and surface variability

Dynamic Leaping & Landing
(e.g., bounding across river rocks or boulders)

- Trains eccentric loading and reactive power

- Demands stabilization and re-acceleration on unstable landings

Pop-Up & Swing-Up Techniques
(e.g., scaling a wall or ledge)

- Develops explosive coordination between the upper and lower body
- Challenges vertical *and* horizontal force production in unpredictable vectors

Heavy Asymmetrical Lifts & Throws
(e.g., hoisting sandbags, logs, or awkward objects overhead)

- Trains raw power with uneven loads and unstable grips
- Requires micro-adjustments with every rep—no two lifts feel the same

Why It Matters

- Explosive strength becomes *omnidirectional*, not just vertical.
- Motor pattern *variability* is preserved, protecting against technical fragility.
- Balance and timing become *responsive*, not rehearsed.

It's one thing to be powerful when every variable is controlled; it's another to be powerful when *nothing* is guaranteed.

Natural movement builds explosiveness that doesn't just shine on a platform—
it succeeds when:

- the ground shifts
- the branch bends
- the wall crumbles

Because the real world won't ask you for a perfect lift.
It will ask if you can respond with power, *no matter the conditions.*

That's adaptive power.
And that's what life demands.

CrossFit: Work Capacity vs. Real-World Wisdom

CrossFit broke the mold—and deserves credit for it.
It shattered the isolationist mindset of single-muscle, single-plane fitness.

It introduced millions to:

- Compound lifts
- Gymnastics skills
- Metabolic conditioning
- Community-driven motivation

CrossFit celebrated work capacity—
the ability to produce high effort across multiple time domains and diverse movement patterns.

That's real.
That's admirable.
It was a massive leap forward from the mirror-bound world of isolated curls.

But CrossFit didn't fully reconnect movement to its biological and ecological roots.

Instead of training for adaptive, environmental problem-solving,
it often substituted randomization for relevance:

- WODs are designed for intensity, not context.
- Complex lifts are performed under fatigue, compromising form and sensorimotor precision.
- Fatigue is pursued as a goal, regardless of its functional transfer.

The result?

- Incredible toughness
- Solid general fitness
- But missing the final layer: movement intelligence that solves real-world challenges

What CrossFit Builds Well

- **Work Capacity –** High-output performance across a range of movement tasks
- **Metabolic Flexibility –** Resilience in switching between energy systems under stress
- **Community Resilience –** Emotional grit through shared suffering and social cohesion

Where CrossFit Falls Short

- **Randomization Over Adaptation** – Random tasks build general fitness but lack contextual learning
- **Technique Erosion Under Fatigue** – High-rep Olympic lifts under exhaustion compromise motor patterns
- **Sensory Calibration Neglect** – Little exposure to unstable surfaces, friction shifts, or real-world object dynamics
- **Over-Glycolytic Bias** – Overreliance on high-intensity effort at the cost of sustainable, intelligent movement

The result?

A body—and a mind—conditioned to suffer,
but not always conditioned to *solve*.

- The barbell doesn't slip.
- The ground doesn't shift.
- The obstacle doesn't think back.

CrossFit hardens the body.
But the world demands more than *hardness*.
It demands a kind of softness: adaptability.

Random endurance is admirable.
Strategic, adaptive endurance is indispensable.

Natural Movement Response: Capacity with Context

Natural movement takes the best of CrossFit—
high work capacity, functional movement, and resilience under

fatigue—
and roots it back in the real world.

Not randomized tasks.
Context-driven challenges.

Key Natural Movements That Parallel—and Surpass—CrossFit Outcomes:

Variable Load Carries
(e.g., transporting stones, logs, or sandbags over uneven terrain)

- Builds full-body endurance, grip resilience, and postural control
- Adapts to shifting loads, terrain irregularities, and changing leverage

Reactive Crawling & Scrambling
(e.g., moving across jagged terrain or unstable slopes)

- Trains cardio and stamina *while* enhancing proprioceptive calibration and environmental coordination
- Builds real-time responsiveness under threat and fatigue

Flow-Based Movement Chains
(e.g., vault → crawl → climb → balance in unpredictable sequences)

- Develops metabolic endurance through integrated skill chaining
- Requires constant perception, decision-making, and creativity, not rote repetition

Rescue Simulations
(e.g., dragging or carrying a person across varied terrain)

- Cultivates strength, endurance, strategy, and emotional resilience under pressure
- Trains *why* we move, not just how

Why It Matters

- Metabolic conditioning is developed through *movement solutions*, not arbitrary exhaustion
- Creativity and decision-making are preserved under fatigue
- Joint and sensory systems are *co-trained*, reducing repetitive strain and injury risk

Random intensity builds toughness.
Contextual intensity builds capability.

Natural movement doesn't merely test your energy systems; it also teaches you to think, feel, and adapt under pressure while still developing the same engines that CrossFit aimed to cultivate.

Because surviving a storm, crossing a river, or rescuing another human will never be *"for time."*

It will be for life.

Training for Stress
How Your Workout Shapes Your Nervous System

Most people consider training in terms of calories burned, muscles developed, or endurance improved. But every workout achieves more than that:

It instructs your nervous system **on** how to interpret and respond to the world.

Lactate and the Language of Stress

At rest, blood lactate levels hover around 1–2 mmol/L— a quiet background hum.

During intense efforts—sprints, heavy lifts, high-intensity intervals—
lactate can spike to 6, 8, even 20 mmol/L.
This isn't dangerous.
It's how your body handles extreme energy demands.

But here's the key:
Lactate isn't just a fuel byproduct.
It's a **stress signal**.

Research shows:

- Lactate rises during emotional stress, not just physical effort
- Elevated lactate correlates with increased **sympathetic activation** ("fight or flight")
- Repeated lactate spikes may influence how your **brain interprets pressure**, even outside the gym

Train High-Intensity All the Time → React Intensely All the Time

If your workouts constantly flood your system with high lactate and sympathetic stress:

- Your body starts to associate effort with **urgency**
- Your brain gets faster at triggering *fight* responses, even to minor challenges
- You begin to carry the signature of crisis into everyday life

That means a program based solely on intensity may unintentionally train you to respond to emotional, social, and professional stress with the same biochemical reaction as fleeing from a predator:

Explosive.
Reactive.
Exhausting.

Natural Movement: Training for Nervous System Literacy

Natural movement still builds capacity—
but through **adaptive**, **context-driven** tasks that require presence, not panic:

- Lifting awkward loads across unpredictable terrain
- Crawling and climbing through unstable environments
- Flowing through movement chains that demand attention, creativity, and patience

And crucially, intensity isn't random—the task regulates it:

- Vaulting a log? High-output burst
- Crawling under branches? Sustained mid-level effort
- Balancing across a fallen tree? Calm, breath-led focus

This organic cycling of intensity teaches your nervous system:

- When to surge
- When to recalibrate
- When to recover without collapsing

Where high-intensity models train fight-or-flight, natural movement encourages graded resilience: a living, responsive readiness that adapts to the moment.

Why It Matters

The way you train is the way you live.
You are teaching your nervous system every time you move.

You can train it to:

- Spike high and crash... or
- Surge, adapt, recover, and move forward with clarity.

Training for life isn't just about what you can endure.
It's about how wisely you respond when pressure arrives.

Natural movement doesn't just build fitness.
It builds freedom.

When Performance Outpaces Physiology: Insulin Resistance in Elite Athletes

It's easy to assume that the more active you are, the healthier you become.
More sweat.
More strain.
More fitness.
Right?

Not always.

Emerging research indicates that **excessive activity-related stress—particularly when combined with insufficient recovery—can result in a paradoxical outcome: insulin resistance.**

Yes—**even in elite athletes.**

This isn't just a CrossFit issue.
It's been observed in:

✦ High-level sprinters

✦ Ultra-endurance athletes

✦ Military trainees

✦ Recreational athletes with high stress + high output + poor recovery

It's what some researchers call **"metabolic rigidity."**
The body becomes **locked in stress chemistry**, even at rest.

Here's how it happens:

- Chronic high-intensity training repeatedly activates the **sympathetic nervous system**.

- This leads to **elevated cortisol** and **glucagon**, both of which oppose insulin.

- **Lactate**, normally a helpful byproduct of energy production, becomes elevated at rest, signaling persistent metabolic strain.

- Recovery is neglected or insufficient: glycogen isn't fully replenished, inflammation builds, and sleep suffers.

- Over time, the body starts to show signs of **impaired glucose tolerance and insulin resistance**, despite visible fitness.

This isn't just about "overtraining."
It's about a **mismatch between stress and recovery**, between output and integration.

The red flags?

- Elevated resting heart rate
- Chronically poor sleep
- Fatigue despite high fitness
- Unexpected weight gain or blood sugar instability
- Constant need for stimulants to get through training

This doesn't mean athletes should avoid intensity.
It means intensity must be **cycled**, **contextualized**, and **recovered from**.

Because the goal is not to be endlessly "on."
The goal is to be able to shift gears:

- Surge when needed
- Recover when possible
- Adapt across the full spectrum of human stress

That's metabolic intelligence.
That's physiological freedom.

You can train for mirrors.
You can train for medals.
You can train for numbers that impress strangers on the internet.

And there's nothing inherently wrong with any of it.
There is real beauty in discipline, in effort, in the pursuit of heavier lifts, faster times, sharper lines.

But if you zoom out—
beyond the gym walls,
beyond the platforms, the chalk, the competition lights—
you'll find a different question waiting for you:

Does your training prepare you for life?

Not just for a barbell.
Not just for a race.
Not just for a stage.

But for:

- The slip on a rocky trail
- The fallen tree blocking your path
- The unexpected sprint to catch a child before they fall

- The hard conversation
- The moment that tests your body, your mind, and your spirit—all at once

Because life doesn't ask how much you can deadlift.
It asks:

- How do you move when the ground shifts beneath you?
- What happens when the plan falls apart?
- Does your strength bend—or break—when real pressure comes?

Training isn't just about building muscle.
It's about building resilience.

It's about shaping a nervous system that knows:

- When to surge
- When to adapt
- When to endure
- When to soften

It's about moving gracefully under pressure.
Thinking clearly despite fatigue. Discovering creativity where others see collapse.

This is the physiology of purpose.

This is the natural kind of movement that doesn't just complement life—
It defends it.

PHYSIOLOGY OF PURPOSE

It honors it.
It expands it.

Train for the unknown.
Train for the uneven ground.
Train for the wildness that made you.

Train not just to survive—
but to meet life's most challenging moments
with a body—and a mind—prepared to move.

This is the path Natural Movement offers.

It's not fitness.
It's not sport.

It's freedom.

The goal of this chapter is not to critique CrossFit, power-lifting, or bodybuilding. Rather, it's to show that **all these training modalities fall under the broader umbrella of natural movement,** they're just specialized expressions of it.

The core message is about adaptability vs. specialization:

- **Are you practicing a wide array of techniques to build well-rounded capability?**
- **Or are you narrowing your physical expression in ways that limit adaptability?**

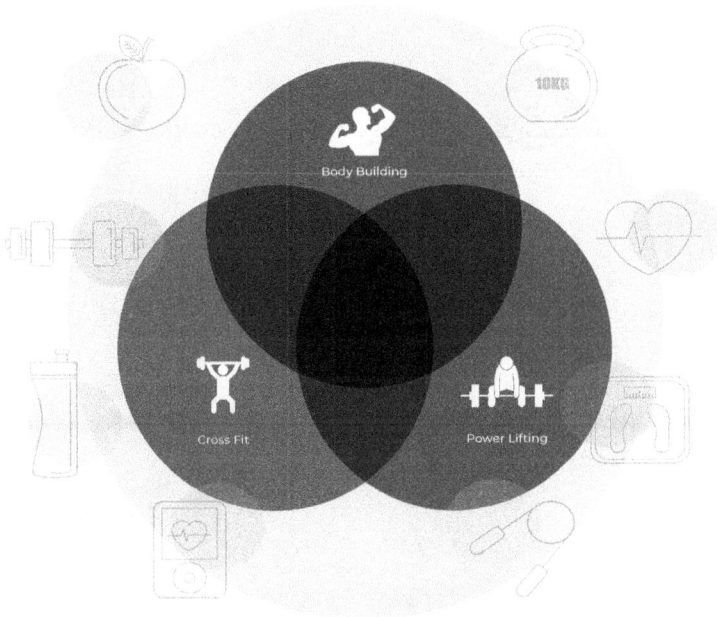

The Physiology of Purpose

Move like it matters.
Because inside you, it always does.

Movement made the brain.
Movement refines the brain.
Movement preserves the brain.

Movement is awareness made real.
Awareness becomes action.
Action becomes survival.

Survival leads to recovery.
Recovery leads to adaptation.
Adaptation leads to freedom.

Freedom is the ability to engage with the world—
not as you wish it were,
but as it is—
and navigate through it gracefully.

Across every stage of life—
you move to become who you are meant to be.

Movement tests the body.
Movement reveals the soul.

CHAPTER 7

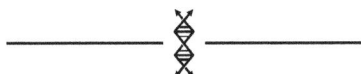

THE RECOVERY OF TRUST PAIN, MOVEMENT, AND HEALING THE BODY

The Injury

It happened fast—
but not recklessly.
Not with malice.

There was no rage in the roll.
No warning siren.
Just the natural chaos of two bodies—
testing, adapting, trying to outthink, outmove, and outfeel
each other.

PHYSIOLOGY OF PURPOSE

Training.
Learning.
Becoming better.

Until it no longer felt that way.

A scramble—
A planted foot—
A slight twist—
A shift in pressure—
pop.

No searing pain.
Just a moment of dissonance.
A quiet realization that something inside him had moved
in a way it was not meant to move.

He sat up slowly, waving off concern from his partner.
Tried to stand.

The knee buckled—
not from pain,
but from betrayal.

A part of him that had always been there—reliable, strong,
unquestioned—
was suddenly gone.

And with it, something deeper slipped away:
Trust.

He limped to the sidelines, heart pounding—
not from exertion,
but from fear.

The room spun—
not from dizziness,
but from disorientation.

How do you move forward
when the body you trusted
no longer answers you?

The injury would later have a name—
ACL tear, meniscus damage, and partial disruption of supporting structures.

The diagnosis would be clean.
Clinical.
Precise.

But no MRI or physical exam could capture the real wound:

The break between mind and body.
The sudden, terrifying realization that
movement can fail.
That effort and attention
can still end in vulnerability.

The hardest part of recovery wouldn't be the knee.
It would be rebuilding the relationship between trust,
movement, and self.

And it would take more than surgery, sets, and reps.
It would take a different kind of healing—
a healing that moved.

Inspired by True Pain

The opening story of this chapter—the hiker's injury—is
told through narrative.
But the experience is real.

In September 2020, I injured my knee during a Jiu-Jitsu
session— grappling with a much larger teammate.
I attempted a submission.
He tried to escape.
And my leg made three distinct popping sounds.

The eventual diagnosis?

- ✦ A **Grade 2+ sprain** of the LCL, MCL, and PCL
- ✦ A likely **near-dislocation** of the knee
- ✦ And based on symptoms, probably a **fracture of
  the lateral tibial tuberosity**

There was pain.
But more than that, there was a sense of panic.
Because I was just six weeks away from my MovNat Level
1 and Level 2 certification.

What followed was an urgent, improvised recovery:
Traditional physical therapy.
Blood flow restriction training.
And a self-guided return to natural movement—using the
ground, deep knee positions, and gradual re-integration of
load and complexity.

I passed my certifications in October.
It was a five-day event.
And I probably re-injured my knee in the process.

It would take another eight months to fully recover.
No surgery.
Just persistence.
And still, to this day, my knee feels like it's held together
by floss.

But here's what matters:
I'm still capable.

Most people wouldn't even be aware of the issue.
Not because the tissue is perfect.
But because I've learned what's safe, what's possible, and
what my body can still do.

That's what this chapter is about.

Not perfection.
Not restoration to a previous version of yourself.
But the rebuilding of trust in your body, in movement, and
in your ability to rise again.

Fear-Avoidance and Movement

Injury doesn't just change the body.
It changes **behavior**.
It changes **belief**.
It changes the way you inhabit yourself.

When the hiker tore his knee on the mat,
the damage wasn't just mechanical.
It sent a silent shockwave through his nervous system.

Suddenly, every step, every pivot, every crouch
came wrapped in a quiet question:

"Will this hurt?"
"Will this fail me again?"

Even movements far from the injured site—
a torso twist, a high reach, a slow descent to the ground—
began to feel different.
Threatening.

The body flinched
before the mind even registered concern.

Muscles stiffened.
Joints moved cautiously, inefficiently.

The world shrank.
Movement—once fluid and automatic—
became preemptive.
Guarded.

This is **fear-avoidant behavior** in action.
And it's one of the greatest silent obstacles to true recovery.

The Physiology of Fear-Avoidance

**When fear of pain enters the system, it alters movement at
every level:**

- **Motor Planning:** Movements are pre-programmed for
  safety, not efficiency
- **Muscle Activation:** Co-contraction increases, creating
  rigidity and energy leaks

- **Sensory Processing:** Threat signals dominate, dulling proprioceptive precision
- **Emotional State:** Anxiety associated with basic movement itself

Over time, this builds a vicious cycle:

- *Fear leads to guarded movement*
- *Guarded movement creates dysfunctional patterns*
- *Dysfunctional patterns reinforce inefficiency and real pain*
- *Pain confirms the original fear*

It's the neuromuscular version of the dark side:

"Fear leads to anger. Anger leads to hate. Hate leads to suffering." —Yoda

Here, it's:

"Fear leads to guarding. Guarding leads to dysfunction. Dysfunction leads to pain. Pain leads to avoidance."

And the more that avoidance takes hold,
the more we forget what freedom ever felt like.

How Natural Movement Breaks the Cycle

Natural Movement principles don't just rebuild strength; they rebuild the relationship between you and your body.

Because Natural Movement doesn't treat movement as isolated exercises.
It treats movement as exploration.

- Ground movement reintroduces bodyweight load gently, re-teaching trust in support structures (hands, knees, hips)
- Crawling and flow work lower threat levels, allowing movement to re-expand without triggering fear responses
- Low-intensity balance work challenges stability while embedding safety through constant micro-corrections
- Play-based movement transforms fear into curiosity— an emotional reframe essential for true healing

Movement doesn't just repair the body.
It retrains the mind to believe in the body again.

Because the real recovery after injury isn't just physical.
It's emotional.
It's neurological.
It's existential.

**To move again freely,
you must believe again deeply.**

Neural Remapping After Injury

Pain is not just a signal.
It's a sculptor.

It reshapes the brain.
It rewires the body's sense of itself.

After the hiker's injury,
something changed inside him—
something deeper than swelling, bruising, or instability.

The map of his body—the internal representation built from years of movement, sensation, and coordination—had become distorted.

The injured knee wasn't just weaker.
It was now different in the brain's perception.
Less certain.
Less "there."

This phenomenon has a name:
Neural Remapping.
And it's one of the most difficult hidden challenges in injury recovery.

The Science of Neural Remapping

The brain maintains detailed **sensory-motor maps** of the body.
These maps enable:

- Smooth coordination
- Accurate proprioception
- Predictive movement planning

But injury disrupts the input:

- **Pain** clouds sensory clarity
- **Immobilization** shrinks feedback loops
- **Fear** reweights signals, amplifying threat and muting exploration

Over time, without movement,
the **neural representation** of the injured area begins to

atrophy—
just like the muscles themselves.

The result?

Even after the tissues heal,
movement can still feel awkward, guarded, or wrong.

Because what's healing isn't just the knee—
it's the **idea** of the knee inside the brain.

How Natural Movement Repairs the Map

Natural Movement isn't just physical rehabilitation; it's
neuro-rehabilitation.

Because it does what rigid, repetitive rehab often fails to do:
it reawakens the brain's *relationship* with the body through
complexity, variability, and play.

Variability of Sensory Input
Crawling, climbing, balancing, carrying—
each delivers rich, diverse streams of feedback
to rebuild sensory clarity and proprioceptive precision.

Task-Oriented Movement
Navigating over, under, and around real obstacles
requires the brain to reconnect intention with execution—
to sync the plan with the experience.

Playful Exploration
Low-threat environments, like ground flow sequences—
give the nervous system space to re-expand its maps
without fear of shutting them down.

Multi-Planar Engagement
Natural Movement isn't linear.
It re-trains the brain to move, think, and predict in the face of unpredictability.
Across the real.

Because movement isn't just mechanical.
It's cognitive.
It's perceptual.
It's how the body teaches the brain to remember itself again.

Healing isn't just about fixing tissue.
It's about restoring identity—
through movement.

Neural Remapping After Injury
How the Brain Rebuilds the Body Map

Movement doesn't start in the muscles.
It starts in the brain—
in intricate, dynamic maps that represent your body's shape, position, and potential actions.

When injury strikes, these maps get distorted.
And recovery isn't just about healing tissue.
It's about helping the mind remember the body—accurately, completely, and confidently.

The Brain's Mapmakers

Several key brain regions work together to create, update, and refine your internal model of movement:

Brain Region	Role
Primary Somato-sensory Cortex (S1)	Receives touch, pressure, and proprioceptive input; forms the "homunculus"—the brain's sensory body map.
Primary Motor Cortex (M1)	Initiates voluntary movement and sends motor commands outward.
Posterior Parietal Cortex	Integrates sensory input (vision, touch, proprioception) for movement planning and spatial awareness.
Cerebellum	Refines movement accuracy, predicts consequences, and supports motor learning.
Insular Cortex	Monitors interoception—internal sensations like heartbeat, breath, and internal tension.

These regions don't operate in isolation.
They constantly cross-reference and recalibrate based on what you feel, intend, and experience.

That's why after an injury, rehab isn't just mechanical.
It must be multi-sensory, task-rich, and emotionally safe—
to invite the brain to rebuild the body map fully.

Injury Disrupts the Maps

When a part of the body is injured, the brain's internal representation of that region begins to degrade.

- **Sensory input decreases**—due to swelling, pain inhibition, and immobility
- **Motor output becomes distorted**—from guarding, compensation, and weakness

- **Feedback loops weaken**—less movement means less sensory updating

In effect, the brain begins to "forget" that part of the body.

Functional MRI studies show that after injuries like ACL tears, wrist fractures, or ankle sprains, the affected area's representation in the primary sensory (S1) and motor (M1) cortices becomes blurred, shrunk, or less active.

This explains why, even after the joint "heals,"
movement may still feel awkward, disconnected, or unstable.

It's not just the joint.
It's the map that needs to heal, too.

Natural Movement: Rewriting the Body's Story

Traditional rehab often focuses on isolated strength or joint-specific range of motion.
These help—
but they rarely rebuild the integrated, sensory-rich maps that real movement demands.

Natural Movement does because it naturally:

- **Challenges proprioception**—balancing, shifting, reaching, adapting
- **Demands sensory integration**—blending touch, pressure, vision, and vestibular input
- **Stimulates interoception**—reconnecting to breath, heartbeat, and tension states
- **Promotes exploration**—inviting the nervous system to rediscover the body's possibilities without fear

Every crawl.
Every vault.
Every awkward lift across shifting ground—

—isn't just rebuilding strength.
It's repainting the body in the brain.

It's teaching the mind:

"This is your body again.
You can trust it.
You can move through the world freely once more."

Rethinking Injury—Three Ways to Understand What Went Wrong

When discussing injury, the explanation matters.
Because how we explain it shapes how we recover from it.

Let's look at three ways people interpret the same event:

1. The Traditional Mechanical View

- Injury is explained by structure and force: *"The knee went into valgus under high load, the ACL couldn't handle the torque."*
- Focus is on external load exceeding tissue tolerance
- The solution? Protect, immobilize, rebuild the tissue

Useful for diagnostics.
But limited. It treats the body like a machine—parts under stress, parts that fail.

2. The Motor Learning View

✦ Injury is explained as a failure of movement behavior under pressure: *"The system lacked a viable solution for the problem the environment presented."*

✦ It's not just about poor coordination— it's about insufficient adaptability within the available movement repertoire.

✦ The body didn't fail because it was weak or slow. It failed because it didn't have enough options.

✦ Focus is on perception-action coupling, task variability, and behavioral flexibility. Movement is seen as an ongoing dialogue with the environment.

✦ The solution? Expand the movement vocabulary. Increase exposure to varied contexts. Train adaptability—not just repetition.

This view is more holistic than traditional mechanics. It treats movement as emergent, not pre-programmed. But without a structural understanding of how the body organizes under load (tensegrity), it can still miss why certain solutions fail under force.

3. The Biotensegrity + Motor Learning View (My Perspective)

✦ Injury is a systems failure—a mismatch between structure, perception, and context.

"The body's tensegrity architecture couldn't dynamically adapt under load—because the available solutions were too few, too rigid, or too slow for the problem at hand."

- The issue isn't just weakness or poor coordination. It's a collapse in dynamic integrity—a loss of both *physical adaptability* and *perceptual fluency*.

- Movement didn't break. The system simply ran out of options.

- This view combines:

- **Biotensegrity** – understanding the body as a responsive, load-distributing structure shaped by tension and compression

- **Motor Learning** – recognizing that movement is *problem-solving*, not rote execution

- **Perceptual Ecology** – seeing injury as a failure of the system to *interpret* and *respond to* threat, pressure, or environmental complexity in real time

- The solution? Rebuild the system with: → Natural movement → Variability and unpredictability → Tensional loading across the fascial web → Restoration of trust, perceptual sensitivity, and behavioral range

This view doesn't just ask *"What broke?"*
It asks:
"Why couldn't the system adapt in time?"
"Why were there no safe options left when pressure arrived?"

In this lens, injury is not a failure of the body.
It's a call to expand its possibilities.

What Is Biotensegrity?

Biotensegrity is a revolutionary way of understanding the body—not as a machine of levers and hinges, but as a living, adaptable structure built from tension and compression.

The term was introduced by Dr. Stephen Levin, an orthopedic surgeon who challenged traditional biomechanics by applying the principles of tensegrity (originally from architecture and sculpture) to human anatomy.

In a biotensegrity system:

Bones don't stack like bricks—they float, suspended in a web of tension (fascia, ligaments, muscles)

Muscles don't just pull on bones—they help distribute force through continuous tension lines

Joints don't just hinge—they respond to forces from all directions, not just a single axis

Movement isn't isolated—it's a whole-system response to load, gravity, and intention

When we say an injury is a collapse of dynamic integrity, we're describing a moment when the body's tensegrity structure couldn't adapt in time.

Biotensegrity helps us understand why movement must be trained as a system, **not as disconnected parts.**

Natural Movement reflects this truth. It loads the system across vectors, planes, and environments—the very conditions that rebuild tensegral adaptability.

Proprioceptive Deficits After Injury

Movement begins with knowing where you are.
Without that knowledge,
every step becomes a guess.
Every reach becomes a risk.

After injury, this "knowing"—
this *felt sense* of position and motion—
fractures.

Even if the muscles regain strength,
even if the joint regains flexibility,
something deeper often remains lost.

The Science of Proprioception

Proprioception is your brain's ability to track body position, tension, and movement *without* conscious attention.

It relies on a network of sensory systems:

- **Muscle Spindles**—detect stretch and rate of change within muscles
- **Golgi Tendon Organs**—sense tension at tendons, preventing overload
- **Joint Receptors**—monitor compression, rotation, and joint angle

- **Skin Mechanoreceptors**—provide tactile feedback from contact, friction, and pressure

Together, these systems form a **real-time internal map** of where your body is and where it's going.

When injury disrupts these channels:

- Precision degrades
- Joint stability declines
- Confidence collapses

The brain can no longer predict movement accurately, so it compensates:

- Over-activating some muscles
- Stiffening joints
- Slowing down reaction timing

It's like trying to drive a familiar road at night— **but without headlights.**

Still possible.
But dangerous.
And exhausting.

True recovery doesn't just strengthen muscles.
It reignites sensory intelligence.

Natural Movement does this beautifully—because it reintegrates proprioception into every task:

- Balancing on rails, branches, and narrow surfaces
- Crawling across uneven textures

- Transitioning between quadrupedal and bipedal movement

Stimulates skin, joints, and muscles dynamically:

- Barefoot locomotion on natural surfaces—grass, sand, rock
- Variable load carries using awkward, shifting objects—not symmetrical dumbbells

Forces constant adjustment and recalibration:

- The environment demands attention
- The body must listen
- The brain must relearn to predict, respond, and adapt

Every Natural Movement challenge becomes a quiet conversation between sensation and action:

- *Where am I?*
- *How am I shifting?*
- *How am I staying upright, efficient, and fluid?*

Proprioception isn't rebuilt through memorized drills.
It's rebuilt through living movement—movement that matters.
A kind of movement that asks and listens simultaneously.

Because healing isn't just about returning to motion.
It's about returning to awareness.

Graded Exposure and Functional Recovery

Healing is not a return to yesterday.
It is the construction of something new—
a relationship between **body, brain, and environment**
that honors what was lost,
but is not defined by it.

After injury, the temptation is strong to either:

- Push too hard, too soon
- Protect too much, for too long

Both extremes create new dysfunctions.

- Pushing too hard risks **re-injury**, overwhelming fragile systems still trying to rebuild
- Protecting too long cements **fear, avoidance**, and **sensory decay**

Recovery demands a third way:
Graded Exposure.

What is Graded Exposure?

Graded exposure is the **intentional, gradual reintroduction** of challenge, carefully adjusted to push the system just enough to encourage adaptation, but not so much that it falls into fear or failure.

It's not *"no pain, no gain."*
It's *"no overwhelming threat—steady, honest challenge."*

Each step forward recalibrates:

- The injured tissue's **capacity**
- The nervous system's **confidence**

- The mind's **trust**

Graded exposure works because it teaches safety through **success**, not avoidance.

It doesn't ask the body to be fearless.
It invites the body to **learn**—
through movement, through feedback, through gradual victories.

Natural Movement shines here—because it offers the ideal structure for progressive, intelligent recovery.

Natural Gradients of Difficulty:

- Crawling before balancing
- Low vaulting before jumping
- Carrying awkward loads before sprinting across uneven terrain

Each challenge emerges naturally from the last.

Movements can be modulated by:

- Speed
- Complexity
- Surface
- Load
- Environment

You're never "stuck"—you're always progressing, adapting, adjusting.

Variability Within Repetition:

Even when repeating the same task, such as crawling, no two
repetitions are truly the same.
Subtle differences in limb position, contact, and force sharpen
sensory-motor precision without overloading the system.

Emotional Regulation Through Movement:

Navigating uncertainty.
Adapting smoothly after mistakes.
Regaining balance when thrown off.

These aren't just physical skills.
They're *psychological capacities*—
built through motion, not mindset alone.

In the hiker's recovery,
the journey wasn't a straight line.

There were stumbles.
Moments of fear.
False starts.

But because he reintroduced movement intelligently—
step by step, sensation by sensation—
his body relearned.

Not just to move.
But to move without fear.

Recovery isn't about returning to *old strength*.
It's about building a new strength—
one that includes vulnerability,
but triumphs anyway.

The body can heal faster than the mind.
A ligament can be stitched.

A bone can be set.
A muscle can regrow.

But trust—
that quiet, unquestioned partnership between intention and action—
takes longer.
And without it, recovery remains incomplete.

Injury doesn't just damage tissue.
It leaves behind an **emotional wound**:

- Fear of re-injury
- Doubt in one's capability
- Loss of a previous identity *("I was strong." "I was athletic." "I could always...")*
- Grief for the quiet sense of invincibility that once lived in every movement

These emotions don't just exist in thought.
They live in the **nervous system**.

They show up as:

- Tension
- Hesitation
- Fatigue
- Collapse under pressure

If emotional healing is ignored—
the body may recover structurally,
but the **spirit stays limping**.

After an injury, the nervous system often recalibrates to prioritize protection.
It becomes:

- Faster at detecting threats
- More anxious at baseline
- Quicker to interpret effort or uncertainty as danger

This protective bias is useful in the acute phase.
It keeps you cautious.
Keeps you still long enough to survive.

But if left unchallenged,
it becomes maladaptive.

Instead of moving into life,
the person starts moving away from it.

Muscles may rebuild.
Tissues may heal.
But the movement stays hesitant.
The world stays smaller.

Healing doesn't just mean strengthening the tissue.
It means retraining the self to:

- Explore again
- Trust again
- Risk again

Because recovery isn't complete until you remember how to move toward life again.

How Natural Movement Rebuilds Psychological Resilience

Natural Movement helps heal the unseen wounds by:

Reintroducing Playful Exploration

- Play disarms the fear centers of the brain.
- It invites curiosity back into movement.
- It makes risk feel like discovery, not danger.

Scaling Risk Safely

- Small successes—crawling, balancing, vaulting low obstacles—rebuild self-efficacy.
- Confidence is earned *without* overwhelming the nervous system.

Creating Meaningful Victories

- Solving a real environmental problem—crossing a creek, climbing a rock, regaining balance reignites belief in capability.
- These are not symbolic wins. They are felt truths.

Honoring Patience

- Natural Movement isn't about "winning the workout."
- It's about rebuilding a relationship between self and body—slowly, respectfully, sustainably

In the hiker's recovery,
the hardest milestone wasn't sprinting again.

It was crouching low.
Moving fast.
Trusting his knee to catch him—without thinking about it.

Not demanding permission from fear.
Not negotiating with hesitation.
Just moving.
Just being.

Healing the body takes medicine.
Healing the mind takes movement.

Healing the Command System
How Movement Recalibrates the Nervous System After
Injury

Injury isn't just a blow to the body.
It's a disruption of the command system itself.

The nervous system—
the living intelligence that once sensed, decided, and
moved without hesitation—
now hesitates.
Now second-guesses.
Now protects first and moves second.

True healing means more than mending tissues.
It means recalibrating the entire network of survival,
coordination, and self-trust.

Key Players in the Nervous System Recalibration

System Component	Role in Recovery
Somatic Nervous System	Controls voluntary movement. After injury, precision and fluidity degrade. Natural Movement retrains **deliberate, confident action** through real tasks.
Autonomic Nervous System	Regulates arousal and recovery. Injury often biases the system toward chronic **threat mode**. Breath-led, playful movement restores balance.
Spinal Reflex Arcs	Manage protective reactions (balance, joint stabilization). Injury may dull or over-activate reflexes. Dynamic movement **recalibrates reflex timing**.
Cerebellum	Coordinates timing, fluidity, and error correction. Injury disrupts prediction. Natural Movement restores **adaptive precision** under load and variation.
Insular Cortex	Senses internal states (breath, tension, fatigue). Injury can numb interoception. Breath-driven, ground-based movement **reawakens internal listening**.

Why Movement Is the Medicine

Natural Movement isn't mechanical repetition.
It's dynamic recalibration.

Because it:

- **Demands sensory integration** *How am I balanced? Where is my weight shifting?*
- **Challenges motor control** *How am I sequencing my actions? Can I adjust midstream?*
- **Triggers autonomic shifts** *Am I calm enough to explore? Alert enough to react?*
- **Stimulates interoceptive listening** *What is my breathing telling me? My heartbeat? My tension levels?*

Every obstacle navigated,
every load adjusted,
every unexpected balance correction—
isn't just a physical victory.

It's a neurological reawakening.

Natural Movement Principles in Rehabilitation

Recovery is not a return to the old self.
It is the forging of a new self—
one wiser, more aware, and more adaptable.

Healing through movement must reflect that truth.
Not by retracing old steps—
but by building new pathways: physiological, neurological, psychological.

This is where Natural Movement shines brightest.

Core Natural Movement Principles for True Recovery

1. Variability Over Repetition

Injured systems don't need more monotony.
They need enriched feedback.

Natural Movement constantly varies:

- Surfaces
- Textures
- Directions
- Loads
- Speeds

This variability forces the body to recalibrate on the fly—strengthening coordination, proprioception, and confidence across changing contexts.

2. Sensory-Motor Reintegration

Natural Movement isn't about isolated strength.
It's about the **conversation between sensation and action.**

Practices like barefoot work, ground transitions, and obstacle negotiation reawaken:

- Tactile sensitivity
- Joint positional awareness
- Dynamic balance
- Interoceptive listening (internal states)

This sensory awakening is the secret ingredient behind deep, lasting recovery.

3. Progressive Challenge, Naturally Graded

Natural environments offer **organic progressions:**

- Crawling on smooth floors → crawling on unstable grass
- Balancing on a wide beam → balancing on a narrow rail
- Carrying moderate, awkward loads → carrying heavier, more unbalanced ones

This mirrors the principle of **graded exposure**—
stretching capacity without triggering overwhelm or reactivity.

4. Breath-Led Recovery

The breath is a barometer of threat.
Natural Movement restores breath-centered recovery by:

- Encouraging **nasal breathing** during ground work
- Training **diaphragmatic control** during carries and balances
- Using breath to regulate emotional state during high-demand tasks

Breath bridges the voluntary and involuntary worlds—
and Natural Movement keeps that bridge strong and alive.

Integration in the Hiker's Story

For the hiker, the return wasn't a checklist.
It wasn't "3 sets of 10 quad extensions."

It was crawling again.
Balancing again.
Climbing again.
Carrying again.

Each step, each stumble, each success
wove a new story into his nervous system:

Not *"I am broken."*
But:
"I am rebuilding."
"I can move again."
"I am whole again."

Movement is not just physical therapy.
It is **narrative therapy**.

It writes a new story—
about who you are,
what you can do,
and where you can go.

Natural Movement doesn't just repair injury.
It **restores freedom**.

Movement is more than muscle.
It is **memory**.
It is **meaning**.

When injury strikes, it doesn't just tear tissue—
it tears **trust**.

It fractures the quiet certainty that your body will catch you,
carry you,
protect you.

It leaves **questions** where there used to be **confidence**.

But healing—**true healing**—
isn't just a return to movement.
It is a **return to yourself**.

Natural Movement teaches that recovery isn't found in isolation.
Not in machines.
Not in linear drills.

It's found in the living complexity of real movement:

- Crawling across uneven ground
- Vaulting low walls with new caution—and new courage
- Balancing between risk and stability—inside and outside the body
- Breathing into uncertainty, and choosing movement anyway

Each small victory whispers:

**"You are not fragile.
You are adaptable."**

Each success rewrites the map inside your brain:

**"This is your body.
This is your capability.
This is your life—returned to you through movement."**

Recovery isn't passive.
It's an act of quiet rebellion.

It's the refusal to be defined by damage.
The refusal to let fear write your future.
The refusal to abandon the body you were born to trust.

You heal by moving.
You heal by exploring.

PHYSIOLOGY OF PURPOSE

You heal by remembering—through action—
who you truly are.

The Physiology of Purpose

Move like it matters.
Because inside you, it always does.

Movement made the brain.
Movement refines the brain.
Movement preserves the brain.

Movement is awareness made real.
Awareness becomes action.
Action becomes survival.

Survival gives rise to recovery.
Recovery gives rise to adaptation.
Adaptation gives rise to freedom.

Freedom is the ability to meet the world—
not as you wish it were,
but as it is—
and move through it beautifully.

Across every stage of life—
you move to become who you are meant to be.

Movement tests the body.
Movement reveals the soul.
Movement rebuilds trust.

CHAPTER 8

―――――― ⸙ ――――――

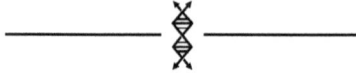

MOVEMENT ACROSS AGING

The forest hadn't changed.
The wind still combed the grass in soft tides.
The sun still spilled gold across the stones.
The trails still wound their quiet paths through the trees.

But **he** had changed.

He crouched at the trailhead, fingertips brushing the earth.
The body that once sprinted across this plain without hesitation now moved with deeper calculation—
not from fear,
but from wisdom.

The knees felt the weight of the years.
The hips whispered reminders of old climbs, falls, and laughter.
The shoulders carried memories of decades—lifting, reaching, throwing, catching.

And yet—

The movement was still there.

He rose smoothly from the crouch,
pressing up through the ground with a strength that was no
longer reckless,
but rooted.

A strength developed not only in muscle,
but over decades of choosing to move, adapt, listen, and grow.

He had not escaped the realities of aging.
The small erosions of time were inevitable.

But he had not surrendered to them, either.

Through movement, he had **negotiated with entropy**—
not by denying the passing years,
but by meeting them with purpose.

And because of that—
he still walked forward into the forest.

Not in defiance of age.
In mastery of it.

Neuromuscular Aging and Energy Systems

Aging does not erase capability. But it asks more of the systems that once operated with effortless resilience.

Now, with every sprint, climb, and reactive movement across uneven terrain, we draw from an energy system that has endured decades of life's challenges.

Understanding how the body's basic energy systems adapt—and decline—with age is crucial for training, movement, and thriving throughout life.

The Changes Beneath the Surface

Movement demands energy.
Energy comes from three primary systems:

- **ATP-PC System**—Immediate energy for explosive efforts
- **Glycolytic System**—Fast anaerobic energy from glucose
- **Oxidative System**—Slow, sustainable energy from fat and glucose

With age, all three adapt—but in different ways.

ATP-PC System: Diminished, But Not Gone

- Creatine phosphate stores decline gradually
- Creatine kinase activity slows, reducing rapid ATP regeneration
- **Result:** Explosive power becomes less available → Jumping across rocks or reacting to a sudden fall feels harder

But the decline isn't absolute.
Through consistent explosive movement—such as vaulting,

crawling sprints, and heavy lifts—the ATP-PC system remains **trainable and resilient**, even into older adulthood.

Glycolytic System and Lactate Dynamics: Subtle Shifts

- Lactate *production* remains relatively stable with age
- Lactate *clearance* slows, especially due to reduced MCT1 and MCT4 transporter expression
- **Result:** Fatigue sets in faster during high-intensity efforts → Tasks like uphill scrambling or extended carrying become more draining

Solution: Train across varied intensities
—not just "go hard," but cycle through moderate, high, and recovery efforts.

Natural Movement does this organically:

- A sprint across a short gap (high lactate burst)
- Followed by climbing or carrying (moderate glycolytic/oxidative blend)
- Then, walking or ground transitions (oxidative recovery)

Nature writes the perfect energy training program—if you listen.

Oxidative System: The Enduring Engine

- Oxygen-based energy remains relatively stable with age, **if movement continues**

- Mitochondrial density and capillary networks do decline, but are highly modifiable

Solution:

- Consistent, task-based movement (hiking, balancing, carrying) preserves mitochondrial function
- Irregular terrain and full-body challenges **stimulate angiogenesis**—the growth of new blood vessels

It's not about endless cardio.
It's about **meaningful, adaptable, consistent movement.**

Integration: Movement as Preservation

When the hiker vaulted a low log,
his ATP-PC system activated with an initial burst.
As he scrambled up the rocky incline,
his glycolytic system took over to support him.
Once he settled into a steady rhythm along the ridgeline trail,
his oxidative system carried him onward.

Age had shifted the balance.
No one system burned as bright as it once had.

But because he kept moving—
training explosiveness, variability, and endurance naturally—
he still had access to the entire orchestra.

The symphony played on.
Not as loud.
But just as powerful.
Just as beautiful.

Fall Risk, Osteopenia, and Postural Control

Aging brings with it many small shifts—
some are almost imperceptible at first:

- A slight hesitation when stepping onto uneven ground
- A barely noticeable wobble when pivoting quickly
- A subtle cautiousness around descents, curbs, and stairs

And then, for many, it brings something bigger:

The fear of falling.

Not because of clumsiness.
But because the systems that once caught you instinctively—
the balance reactions, the bone resilience, the postural
reflexes— have grown slower, weaker, or more brittle.

Sarcopenia Is Not Destiny

Sarcopenia is the age-related loss of muscle mass and strength. It typically begins around the age of 30 and accelerates after 60— with older adults losing up to 3–8% of muscle mass per decade.

But here's what often gets missed:

- Muscle **power** declines **faster** than strength
- Sarcopenia isn't just about shrinking muscles—it's about shrinking **movement capacity**
- The decline is **not inevitable**—it's highly modifiable through intelligent, full-body movement

Traditional strength training can help.
But Natural Movement goes further:

- It loads the body across planes, postures, and patterns
- It improves **motor recruitment**, **coordination**, and **postural integrity**
- It stimulates **myofascial remodeling** and **joint resilience**, not just hypertrophy

You don't beat sarcopenia with sets and reps.
You beat it by moving like life still demands something from you.
Because it does.

The Hidden Architecture Behind Balance

Balance is not a single sense.
It's the **integration** of multiple systems:

- **Vestibular input** (inner ear sensing head position and motion)
- **Visual input** (tracking movement and maintaining orientation)
- **Proprioceptive input** (joint and muscle position feedback)
- **Postural reflexes** (spinal cord-mediated automatic stability responses)
- **Muscle power** (the ability to react and correct quickly)

With age, all of these systems change:

- Vestibular hair cells **decline in number**
- Visual acuity and depth perception **decrease**
- Proprioceptive acuity **dulls**
- Reaction times **slow by 15–30%**
- Muscle **power** declines faster than strength, reducing rapid correction ability

It's not that older adults lose the desire to move well; it's that the biological structure supporting movement gradually deteriorates—subtly and relentlessly.

Unless it is maintained.
Unless it is challenged.
Intelligently.

The Silent Threat: Osteopenia and Bone Fragility

Alongside neuromuscular decline, another hidden risk grows:

- **Bone mineral density** begins to decline after the third decade of life.

- Osteopenia (low bone density) affects nearly **half of Americans over 50**.

- Untreated, it can progress to osteoporosis— leaving bones brittle, porous, and prone to fracture from even minor falls.

Fractures are not just orthopedic issues.

They are life-altering events:

- 1 in 3 adults who fracture a hip never regain full independence.

- Fracture risk **doubles** every decade after 50 without preventive action.

Bones, like muscles, respond to stress—
but only if it is the right kind of stress.

Natural Movement: The Antidote to Fragility

Natural Movement uniquely strengthens the entire fall-prevention architecture:

- **Proprioceptive Training:** Crawling, balancing, ground transitions, and unstable surfaces help maintain sharp joint-position sense.

- **Reactive Stability:** Dynamic carries, obstacle negotiation, multi-planar shifts, and retrain fast, powerful corrections.

- **Bone Loading:** Carrying uneven loads, bounding, crawling under load—all stimulate osteogenesis (bone-building processes) through multi-angled, natural mechanical stress.

- **Cognitive-Motor Integration:** Problem-solving movements (vaulting, navigating terrain) maintain quickness of mind and body coordination.

- **Fear Reconditioning:** Exposure to low-threat imbalances (e.g., crawling on uneven grass, balancing on low beams) rewires fear circuits, reducing the catastrophic fear of falling.

Integration into the Hiker's Story

At 65, the hiker still wasn't immune to instability.
He could still trip. The ground could still move.
The unexpected still occurred.

But his body knew how to catch itself.

His joints whispered real-time reports to his brain.
His muscles reacted with practiced speed.
His bones—dense and prepared—absorbed shock without breaking.

He did not move like a reckless youth.
He moved like a human who had trained **adaptability over time**.

And that made all the difference.

Cognitive-Motor Integration

Aging is often framed as a battle against physical decline:
Muscle mass.
Bone density.
Reaction time.

But beneath all of that—there's another erosion, quieter and far more devastating if left unchallenged: the deterioration of **cognitive-motor integration**.

What Is Cognitive-Motor Integration?

Every movement you make isn't just a muscle firing.
It's a conversation between:

- *Sensation*
- *Perception*
- *Memory*
- *Prediction*
- *Execution*

Examples of this silent dialogue:

- *Seeing an obstacle → predicting how to adjust your stride → executing the adjustment*
- *Feeling a shift in surface → recalibrating posture → preserving balance*
- *Remembering past patterns → applying them creatively in new situations*

This is **cognitive-motor integration**: the unseen dance between brain and body that enables you to move smoothly through the world.

And with every passing decade, it matters more.

How Aging Affects This Dance

- **Neural conduction velocity slows**
- **Processing speed declines**
- **Multisensory integration** (e.g., visual + vestibular + proprioceptive) becomes less efficient
- **Working memory**, the ability to hold and manipulate information, shrinks
- **Attention control weakens**, especially under dual-task or physical stress

The result?

- Movements become slower, less coordinated, and more effortful
- **Dual-task challenges**—walking while talking, stepping while scanning terrain—become dramatically harder
- **Fall risk, injury likelihood, and functional loss** increase sharply

But—this decline is not inevitable.

*The nervous system remains **plastic across life.***
It can adapt.
It can rewire.
If it is challenged the right way.

Natural Movement isn't just physical.
It is inherently **cognitive.**

Because it:

Demands real-time problem-solving
Every terrain shift, every unstable surface, every obstacle
requires **split-second decisions.**

Challenges dual-tasking naturally
Balance while scanning.
Vault while planning.
Carry while navigating.

Enhances multisensory integration
Proprioception, vestibular sense, vision, tactile feedback—
all must **coordinate fluidly under stress.**

**Stimulates memory and prediction—recognizing affordances
in the environment**
Can I step here? Vault there?
Directly taps into motor memory, planning, and creativity.

Every time the hiker crossed a rocky stream,
navigated a fallen tree,
or climbed a steep incline without rails to guide him—he
wasn't just maintaining muscle.

He was preserving his mind.

He was rehearsing **complex, dynamic conversations** between brain and body.
He was preventing the slow, creeping silence
that settles in when movement becomes mechanical,
cautious,
narrow.

The Battle Against Entropy

Aging is often framed as a failure.
A loss.
A decline.

But if you look closer, beneath the fearmongering headlines and shallow slogans, you see something deeper:

Aging is entropy.
And movement—
true, dynamic, living movement—
is resistance.

What Is Entropy?

In simple terms, entropy is the universal drift toward disorder.

- Structures decay
- Energy dissipates
- Complexity collapses into randomness

Biology fights a lifelong war against this tide:

- Cells organize energy into tissue and form
- Systems coordinate action with astonishing precision
- The nervous system orchestrates motion and adaptation in real time

But this battle isn't static. It's ongoing. From conception to the last breath, life continually fights to keep order against the universe's pull toward chaos.

How Aging and Entropy Intertwine

As biological systems age:

- Mitochondria falter, reducing cellular energy
- Muscle fibers atrophy, losing density and structure
- Bone matrix degrades, becoming porous and fragile
- Neural networks weaken, losing synaptic strength and efficiency

All of it is entropy.
Not failure.
Not weakness.
Just nature's most ancient, most persistent law at work.

But within the human body, there exists something extraordinary: the ability to fight back.

The ability to reimpose order,
to restore complexity,
to adapt again—
through intentional movement.

Natural Movement as the Anti-Entropy Engine

Natural Movement doesn't fight aging.
It fights **entropy**.

It doesn't ignore that time is passing.
It prepares the body and brain to meet it—capable, aware, and resilient.

It trains the system to:

- **Rebuild lost neural pathways** through novel motor learning
- **Stimulate mitochondrial biogenesis** through complex, full-body locomotion
- **Thicken bone and muscle fibers** through load-bearing, multi-directional force application
- **Preserve flexibility, balance, and responsiveness**—the abilities needed to solve unpredictable real-world problems

Every crawl, climb, jump, vault, and carry—every time the hiker moved with **purpose**, **complexity**, and **adaptability**—he was telling entropy:

"You will not have me easily."

He wasn't reversing aging.
He was refining himself against it.

Life Quality Through Movement

It's not enough to survive.
Life demands more.

It demands color.
Curiosity.
Connection.
Creation.

Without these, survival becomes a hollow existence. And movement—**true, capable, dynamic movement**—is one of the great enhancers of life quality over the decades.

How Movement Shapes Life Beyond Health Metrics

Domain	How Movement Sustains It
Autonomy	Rising from the ground. Carrying your own groceries. Walking freely without hesitation or assistance.
Joy and Play	Sprinting toward a grandchild. Climbing a tree. Splashing through a river. Balancing on a beam—just because.
Identity & Dignity	Knowing your body isn't a burden—it's a **trusted partner**, not a prison.
Social Connection	Traveling, hiking, dancing, sharing movement-based experiences—without fear of being left out or left behind.
Emotional Resilience	Physical capability reinforces mental strength. Movement becomes a daily reminder that **growth never stops**.

Movement isn't just about **avoiding decline** or staying out of a nursing home.

It's about chasing sunsets across beaches at 65.
It's about crouching low to plant a garden—without groaning—at 70. It's about vaulting a fallen branch at 75 because your soul wanted to feel weightless again.

It's about being able to say **"yes"** to life's invitations instead of **"no"** because your body has become a burden—something to carry vs something you *are*.

Natural Movement as a Lifelong Companion

Natural movement isn't fake. It's not a trendy gym routine that becomes meaningless over time. It is the essential human language.

- Crawl
- Balance
- Climb
- Run
- Vault
- Carry
- Swim
- Jump
- Throw
- Catch

It's every archetypal expression of what it means to inhabit a human body—
kept alive, kept refined, kept joyful across every decade.

You don't *outgrow* Natural Movement.
It grows with you.

It becomes less about conquering records,
and more about expanding experience.

In the hiker's 65-year-old stride,
there was no desperation.
No clinging to lost youth.

There was only **capability**, adapted across seasons.
There was only the pure, simple, enduring joy—
of still being able to move through the world
on his own terms.

Movement Is the Long Game

There is no stopping the seasons.
No denying the slow, inevitable changes that come with time.

The hair turns gray. The skin becomes thinner.
The reflexes slow down.
The body responds to the whispers of entropy.

But inside you—inside every person who dares to move, adapt, and reach—
there is something the years cannot take away.

There is the **choice** to cultivate resilience.
There is the **power** to preserve dignity.
There is the **joy** of a body still capable of exploring the world—
of feeling the rush of breath,
the strength of limbs,
the elegance of balance.

You are not fighting aging.
You are writing your answer to it.

Movement is not the denial of age.
It is the **fulfillment** of it.

It is standing in the face of time and saying:

> "I will not become a prisoner inside my own body.
> I will not retreat from life.
> I will continue to reach, to lift, to leap, to breathe—

because movement is life,
and I am still alive."

Movement is the **language of freedom**.
The **architecture of resilience**.
The **celebration of existence** itself.

Grow older.
Grow wiser.
But never stop moving.

Because the body that moves is the body that lives.
And the soul that moves
is the soul that continues
to sing.

The Physiology of Purpose

Move like it matters.
Because inside you, it always does.

Movement made the brain.
Movement refines the brain.
Movement preserves the brain.

Movement is awareness made real.
Awareness becomes action.
Action becomes survival.

Survival gives rise to recovery.
Recovery gives rise to adaptation.
Adaptation gives rise to freedom.

Freedom is the ability to meet the world—
not as you wish it were,
but as it is—
and move through it beautifully.

Across every stage of life—
you move to become who you are meant to be.

Movement tests the body.
Movement reveals the soul.
Movement rebuilds trust.
Movement transcends aging.

CHAPTER 9

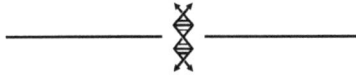

THE NERVOUSE SYSTEM, STESS AND RECOVERY

The Invisible Predator

The wolves were long gone.
The forest paths had been paved for city streets.
The smell of exhaust and concrete replaced the sharp scent of pine and stone.

The dangers were no longer teeth and claws.
Now, the danger was time.

Deadlines.
Expectations.
Unspoken resentments.
Flickering screens.
Endless scrolling.
Sleepless nights under low ceilings instead of stars.

PHYSIOLOGY OF PURPOSE

The world had changed.
But the body had not.

It still watched.
Still waited.
Still tensed.

The heart still raced.
The pupils still widened.
The lungs still flooded—
not from sprinting across open ground,
but from reading an email at 11:42 p.m.
From sitting in a meeting where the air felt heavier than the words.
From wondering—always wondering—if safety was just an illusion now.

The body had once been a chariot of freedom.
Now, for many, it had become a theater of silent war.

But inside him—inside the man who had spent his life moving, adapting, listening to the old songs of his biology—something different stirred.

He remembered.

He remembered how the body fights for life.
How it signals danger and survival.
How it pleads for movement, for action, for resolution.

He remembered that **stress was never the enemy**.
Stagnation was.

And he knew—if he was to live well in this new world,
he had to honor the body's ancient commands in a modern landscape.

He had to move.
Not to **escape**.
But to **restore**.

Sympathetic Activation—When Survival Goes Awry

The sympathetic nervous system is often referred to as the
"fight or flight" system.
But that phrase doesn't capture its full majesty.

It's not just a panic button; it's an ancient orchestra, finely
tuned to a singular purpose:

Survive.

- Blood vessels constrict to redirect flow to the muscles.

- The heart hammers faster, pushing oxygen-rich blood outward.

- Pupils dilate, taking in more light, sharpening the edges of the world.

- The liver floods the bloodstream with glucose for rapid energy.

- The adrenal glands release cortisol—the readiness hormone—priming every cell for war.

The body becomes a spear hurled forward by evolution.
It is beautiful.
It is powerful.
It is necessary.

But it was never meant to be constant.

The Modern Hijacking

In the wild, the stress response was **short-lived**:

You **fought**.
You **fled**.
You **froze**.
You **hid**.
You **healed**.

Then it ended.

But modern life doesn't give clean endings.

Deadlines don't chase you through the forest; they sit in your inbox, gnawing, unresolved, forever pending.

Arguments don't end with a sprint to safety; they echo in text messages,
in worried dreams,
in silent, simmering glances across a dinner table.

The sympathetic system stays primed.
And the human body—designed for action—begins to decay under inaction and chronic tension.

- Heart rate remains elevated
- Breath becomes shallow
- Muscles stay subtly braced
- Glucose remains high
- Inflammation creeps upward
- Recovery systems stay suppressed

You were built to survive wolves.
But now, it is the wolves you never see that wear you down.

Natural Movement as an Antidote

Intelligent, variable movement acts as a reset button.

- **Dynamic motion** discharges sympathetic energy in a safe, embodied way.
- **Load-bearing and locomotion** signal to the nervous system that the threat has passed.
- **Varied physical tasks** retrain the body to shift gears fluidly, rather than remaining stuck in fight-or-flight mode.

Movement—when done with awareness and variability—doesn't just burn calories.

It rewires survival
back into vitality.

Parasympathetic Recovery—The Skill of Rebuilding Calm

Recovery is not the absence of stress.
It's not a passive return to baseline.
 It's not collapsing on the couch and hoping your nervous system fixes itself.

Recovery is a skill—
a dynamic, living ability to shift gears, to re-balance,
to rebuild the internal terrain after activation.

The **parasympathetic nervous system** is the architect of that skill.

What the Parasympathetic System Does

When the parasympathetic system activates:

- **Heart rate slows**, easing the cardiovascular load.
- **Blood vessels dilate**, nourishing tissues with oxygen-rich blood.
- **Breathing deepens**, feeding the brain and body with restorative air.
- **Digestive processes resume**, supporting repair and energy replenishment.
- **Inflammation resolves**, clearing cellular debris and restoring balance.
- **Hormonal cascades shift**, moving toward growth, recovery, and regeneration.

If the **sympathetic system is the warrior**, and the **parasympathetic system is the healer**.

They are not enemies.
Opposite one another, but not opposed.
They are **partners in a dance**.
Yin and yang.

If you cannot recover, **you cannot truly survive**.

Why Recovery Is a Trainable Skill

Modern life doesn't just **overstimulate** the sympathetic
system.
It **atrophies** the parasympathetic.

- Chronic stress trains **shallow, rapid breathing.**
- Sedentary behavior desensitizes the body's sensors
  for **safety and restoration.**
- Poor movement quality limits the body's ability to
  discharge accumulated tension.

Just as you train **strength**, **balance**, and **endurance—**
you must also train **recovery.**

You must remind the body through breath,
through posture,
through deliberate sensory experience—
that it is safe to rebuild, to grow, and that the storm has
passed.

Tools for Parasympathetic Recovery:

Tool	How It Works
Breathwork	Deep diaphragmatic breathing stimulates the **vagus nerve**, the main parasympathetic highway—shifting the body out of fight-or-flight mode.
Slow, Ground-Based Movement	Crawling, flowing, and low gait patterns engage **proprioceptive and vestibular feedback**, re-centering the body's internal state of safety.
Visual and Auditory Widening	Softening the gaze and tuning into ambient sound helps exit **tunnel vision survival mode** and reopens broad sensory awareness.
Rhythmic Locomotion	Gentle walking—especially in nature—**synchronizes cardiac and respiratory rhythms**, promoting calm and baseline restoration.

When the hiker finished a challenging climb,
he didn't collapse in exhaustion.

He slowed his breathing deliberately.
He expanded his awareness to include the sway of trees and the whisper of wind.
He let the movement gradually decrease, not halt suddenly.

He taught his body, over and over again—
that after effort, there could be peace.

And in doing so, he preserved his capacity to make an effort again.

**Not by grinding harder.
But by recovering smarter.**

Heart Rate Variability (HRV)—Measuring Your Nervous System's Adaptability

If you could peer inside your nervous system,
you wouldn't see a machine humming at constant speed.

You would see rhythm.
Tension and release.
Effort and ease.
Activation and recovery.

The body isn't built for **consistency**.
It's built for **adaptability**.

And one of the clearest ways to see that adaptability is
through a simple, powerful measurement:

Heart Rate Variability.

What Is Heart Rate Variability?

HRV measures the **variation in time between each heartbeat**.

Not your heart rate.
Not beats per minute.

But the **tiny differences between beats**:

- One interval might be **802 milliseconds**
- The next, **811 milliseconds**
- The next, **798 milliseconds**

This variation is a **good** thing.

- **More variability** = a responsive, adaptable nervous system
- **Less variability** = a rigid, stressed system struggling to shift between effort and recovery

Why HRV Matters

High HRV	Low HRV
Flexible nervous system	Stuck in fight-or-flight
Fast recovery from stress	Slow, incomplete recovery
Enhanced cognitive flexibility	Reduced executive function
Resilient emotional regulation	Increased anxiety, emotional fragility

High HRV doesn't mean you're always "calm."
It means you can move gracefully between states:

- Activation when needed
- Recovery when needed

It's not about being mellow.
It's about being adaptive.

HRV is the signature of a healthy, responsive human system.

How to Train for Higher HRV

- **Movement Variety** Engaging in diverse intensities, patterns, and speeds enhances the nervous system's range of adaptability.
- **Breath Control** Slow, rhythmic breathing—especially exhalation-focused—improves HRV by increasing **vagal tone.**

- **Natural Recovery** Walking outdoors, exposure to sunlight, and rhythmic locomotion activate **parasympathetic recovery** pathways.

- **Stress Intelligence** Recognizing sympathetic activation and **consciously shifting** toward recovery—rather than waiting for collapse—builds nervous system resilience.

The hiker's recovery wasn't an accident.
It was the product of years spent training fluidity:

- Sprint when needed.

- Slow when needed.

- Breathe when needed.

- Rest when needed.

He didn't remain trapped in survival mode. He moved past it—because his heart, mind, and lungs were conditioned to dance between tension and relaxation.

HRV wasn't just a number.
It was a fingerprint of capability.
A biological signature of freedom.

Movement, Lactate, and Happiness—The Hidden Chemistry of Resilience

Everyone knows exercise is "good for you."

Doctors say it.
Billboards say it.
Social media screams it.

But almost no one tells you **why** it feels good.
Why do you walk away from a session not just physically spent,
but emotionally lighter, clearer, **more capable?**

The answer isn't just **endorphins.**
It's something deeper.
Something more elegant.
Something almost no one talks about:

Lactate.

Lactate: More Than a Byproduct

For decades, lactate was misunderstood.

Branded as a **waste product.**
Blamed for **fatigue.**
Feared as the **chemical enemy of athleticism.**

But modern science has revealed a different story:

- Lactate is produced naturally during movement, even at moderate intensities.

- It crosses the blood-brain barrier via specialized transporters (**MCT1, MCT2**).

- Inside the brain, it binds to receptors like **HCAR1**, triggering powerful growth pathways.

Lactate doesn't poison the brain.
Lactate feeds it.

Once inside the brain, lactate helps:

- Increase **Brain-Derived Neurotrophic Factor (BDNF)**—the master molecule for learning, memory, and emotional resilience.
- Enhance **neuroplasticity**, allowing faster adaptation to new challenges.
- Enhance **stress resilience**, making you more resilient to life's pressures.

Movement creates lactate.
Lactate tells the brain: Grow. Adapt. Strengthen. Feel alive.

An Emerging Theory
Beyond BDNF and brain fuel, lactate may also support the balance of key neurotransmitters:

- **Dopamine** → motivation, drive, reward
- **Serotonin** → mood regulation, emotional stability
- **GABA** → calmness, emotional buffering against stress

How?

- By providing vital energy to neurons when they need it most
- By buffering metabolic stress and reducing neuroinflammation
- By supporting astrocyte-neuron interactions that sustain neurotransmitter cycling

The theory:
Movement doesn't just "make you feel good."
It may support the **chemical foundations of hope, motivation, and emotional regulation** at the cellular level.

This theory, while biologically plausible and supported by early data, is **still emerging**.
Large-scale clinical trials haven't fully confirmed it.

But the pieces are there.
And the logic flows beautifully:

Movement → Lactate → Brain activation, plasticity, and potentially neurotransmitter resilience.

Why This Changes Everything

Movement isn't just exercise.
It's emotional engineering.
It's neural fertilizer.
It's biochemical hope, made tangible through your own muscles and breath.

Every time you move well, breathe deep, sweat with purpose—you aren't just training muscles.

You're sending messages of:

- Growth
- Joy
- Resilience
- Possibility

into your brain's very chemistry.

The hiker, after every climb, every crawl, every sprint, wasn't just building stronger legs.
He was building a stronger mind.

He was growing new possibilities inside himself,
with every surge of breath, blood, and lactate.

He was reminding his brain:

> "You are built for this.
> You are built to grow.
> You are built to survive—beautifully."

Movement and the Immune System—Training the Body's Inner Defenders

The immune system is often imagined as a fortress wall:
Rigid. Static. Built to repel.

But the reality is far more dynamic.

The immune system is a living, adaptive army—
constantly patrolling, evaluating, evolving.

And like every other system in the body,
it listens to movement.

Every time you move, you send signals deep into your internal terrain:

- Circulation increases, carrying immune cells (like natural killer cells and T-cells) to more areas of the body.

- Moderate movement enhances immune surveillance, facilitating the early detection of pathogens and damaged cells.

- Breath-driven movement maintains mucosal defenses—your first-line immunity in lungs, gut, and sinuses.

- Variable intensity trains inflammatory intelligence—keeping immune responses sharp but not overactive.

Movement isn't just good for your muscles.
It's a form of immune education.

The Stress–Immunity Connection

Earlier, we explored how sympathetic activation prepares the body for survival:

- Cortisol rises
- Catecholamines flood the system (adrenaline, noradrenaline)
- Blood flow is shunted to muscles, away from digestion and deep immune function

In short bursts? Perfect.

But in chronic, low-grade stress—the kind that characterizes modern life—this response turns harmful.

It erodes immunity by:

- Suppressing infection-fighting cells
- Increasing background inflammation (*a process now called "inflammaging"*)
- Slowing recovery from illness and injury

Movement modulates this.

Moderate-intensity movement helps balance cortisol rhythms, preventing both suppression and hyperactivation.

Breath-focused recovery practices stimulate vagal tone, reducing systemic inflammation.

Varied-intensity natural movement mirrors ancient patterns—sprinting when needed, recovering thoroughly afterward—keeping both stress systems and immune defenses tuned, not frayed.

Natural Movement: The Original Immune Training

Why is Natural Movement uniquely suited to immune preservation?

Because its patterns—crawling, climbing, carrying, sprinting, flowing—mimic the natural stress–recovery cycles that biology expects:

- Short bursts of intensity (sprinting, vaulting) → stimulate healthy stress adaptation
- Periods of lower intensity (walking, crawling, balancing) → promote parasympathetic recalibration
- Dynamic engagement with varied environments (outdoor terrain, uneven loads) → challenges multi-sensory processing and immune flexibility

Modern fitness often abuses stress:

"Go hard every day."
"Never stop grinding."

But Natural Movement harmonizes stress and recovery. It restores the immune system's natural rhythm— it's a conversation with life:

- Alert when needed
- Calm when safe
- Capable of adapting, not crumbling

Immunity Isn't Just Defense. It's Intelligence.

Movement doesn't just strengthen the body.
It sharpens the body's inner scouts.
Its sentinels.
Its warriors.

It teaches them:

- When to react
- When to stand down
- How to distinguish a genuine threat from harmless noise

Just as the hiker's body learned to sprint away from danger and recover without collapsing, his immune system learned the same wisdom.

Attack when necessary.
Heal when possible.

Breath, Perception, and Recovery—Mastering the Nervous System's Dance

Movement initiates the cycle.
Lactate fuels it.
Recovery closes it.

But something else weaves through every stage:
Breath.

Breath is the bridge between intention and instinct.
It is the leverage you always carry—
the key to guiding your nervous system from moment to moment,
effort to recovery, tension to calm.

Breath: The Original Language of Survival

Breath is not passive.
It is an active conversation between:

- The pons and medulla—brainstem centers that regulate breathing
- The lungs and mechanoreceptors—sensing expansion and pressure
- The heart and baroreceptors—monitoring shifts in blood pressure
- The autonomic nervous system—ready to tip toward sympathetic or parasympathetic states based on respiratory input
- When breathing speeds up, the brain interprets a threat.
- When breath slows, the brain interprets safety.

Breath isn't just the fuel for movement.
It is the conductor of experience.

Training Breath as a Nervous System Skill

Mastering breath is not just about breathing slowly all the time.
It's about matching breath to need—
like a skilled conductor setting the tempo to match the score.

Movement Sharpens Breath Awareness

Natural Movement doesn't separate breath from action.

- Crawling demands breath-timed core engagement.
- Climbing challenges involve inhalation against effort and gravity.
- Carrying teaches controlled exhalation under load.
- Flow work softens and harmonizes your respiratory rhythm.

The body doesn't learn breath control from lectures.
It learns through movement under meaningful challenge.
It learns through real engagement with real demands.

The hiker didn't think about his breathing while escaping the wolves.
He didn't consciously slow his breath while crouching after the sprint.

But because he had moved, trained, and practiced recovery over the years—his body knew what to do.

His lungs, heart, brain, and muscles conversed in the ancient
language of survival.
And because he had never stopped honoring that language—

He survived not just the sprint...
but the aftermath.

You are not meant to be calm all the time.
You are not meant to be tense all the time.

You are meant to be fluid—
to move between states,
to rise when needed,
to rest when possible,
to adapt without losing yourself.

This is not a weakness.
This is not fragility.
This is mastery.

The nervous system is not a machine.
It is a living river:
sometimes raging,
sometimes winding,
sometimes still.

You don't control the river by damming it.
You master the river by understanding its currents—
by knowing when to paddle and when to float,
by trusting the flow that has carried life for millions of years.

When you **sprint**, you honor survival.
When you **breathe**, you honor recovery.
When you **move**, you honor the ancient intelligence encoded
in every cell.

When you train adaptability—
through **movement**, **breath**, **recovery**, and **awareness**—
you aren't just exercising your body.

You are refining your ability to **live**.
You are writing **resilience** into your flesh and spirit.

You are dancing the original dance of life:

- Tension and release
- Action and rest
- Fire and stillness
- Strength and surrender

And in that dance, you find the **freedom no stressor can steal.**

The Physiology of Purpose

Move like it matters.
Because inside you, it always does.

Movement made the brain.
Movement refines the brain.
Movement preserves the brain.

Movement is awareness made real.
Awareness becomes action.
Action becomes survival.

Survival gives rise to recovery.
Recovery gives rise to adaptation.
Adaptation gives rise to freedom.

Freedom is the ability to meet the world—
not as you wish it were,
but as it is—
and move through it beautifully.

Across every stage of life—
you move to become who you are meant to be.

Movement tests the body.
Movement reveals the soul.
Movement rebuilds trust.
Movement transcends aging.
Movement becomes a conversation between life and will.

CHAPTER 10

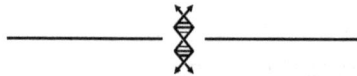

THE RIDGE AND THE RETURN

The trail was steep,
 but not impossible.

He moved carefully now—not out of weakness,
but from presence.

Each step was placed with quiet confidence.
Each breath is drawn with deliberate patience.

The forest behind him blurred into the shadows of memory:
the wolves,
the falls,
the climbs,
the pain,
the triumphs.

Ahead, the world stretched wide and golden.
The sun hung low over the horizon,
casting long amber shadows across the land.

He stood still—
for the first time in what felt like years—
and let the weight of it all settle into his bones.

Movement had once been survival—
sprinting from danger,
crawling from pain,
vaulting over fear.

Movement had once been proof—
of strength,
of ability,
of defiance against entropy.

But now?
Now movement was something else.

It was *belonging*.
It was a return to something ancient and whole:

- The body trusted itself again.
- The mind trusted the body again.
- The spirit trusted life again.

He shifted his weight softly, feeling the small adjustments ripple through his ankles, knees, hips, and spine. He sensed the balance—the communication—the harmony.

Nothing needed to be forced.
Nothing needed to be conquered.

There was no audience.
No timer.
No scoreboard.

PHYSIOLOGY OF PURPOSE

Just the quiet knowledge:

"I am capable.
I am still growing.
I am still alive."

He smiled—
not with triumph,
but with gratitude.

Because movement was no longer just about survival.
It was about trust.
It was about freedom.
It was about coming home.

Movement as Reconnection—Healing the Divide Between Body, Mind, and Life

Injury drives a wedge between you and your body.
So does fear.
So does loss.
So does aging—when the first slow betrayals creep into joints that once felt eternal.

When pain arrives, when movement stalls, when confidence breaks down—a divide emerges.

You lose trust in your body.
And when you stop trusting your body,
a part of you stops trusting yourself.

When injury or trauma strikes,
the **sensory maps** inside the brain begin to blur.

- **Proprioception** (body awareness) degrades.
- **Balance** becomes hesitant.

- **Movement** feels clumsy, dangerous, foreign.

You don't just lose **strength**.
You lose the **sense** of feeling safe within yourself.

Healing is not just about **fixing tissues**.
Healing is about **redrawing the map**.
And the ink... is **movement**.

- **Crawling** rewires forgotten pathways of coordination.
- **Climbing** rebuilds joint confidence and spatial orientation.
- **Walking on varied terrain** restores balance, adaptability, and sensory awareness.
- **Carrying, vaulting, flowing**—each act is a vote of trust, cast from body to mind and back again.

The nervous system **listens**.
The brain **rewrites itself**.
The divide **closes**.

Not all at once.
Not perfectly.
But undeniably.

The hiker didn't regain his body by **thinking**,
 or **waiting**,
 or **hoping**.

He rebuilt it through **living motion**:

- **Testing**—gently, at first
- **Expanding**—cautiously, at first

- **Trusting again**, step by reclaimed step

Trust Is a Skill

Trust Factor	Movement Practice
Self-Perception	Re-engaging sensory systems through mindful, embodied movement
Self-Efficacy	Completing novel or challenging tasks, even imperfectly
Autonomy	Reclaiming daily actions without fear of fragility
Joy	Rediscovering playfulness without guarding, flinching, or overthinking

You don't wait for trust to come back.
You build it.

Through **effort**.
Through **failure**.
Through **curiosity**.
Through the **living, breathing dialogue** between mind and body.

Before you ever said a word,
before you ever had a thought,
your body was already speaking to you.

Through **sensation**.
Through **contact**.
Through **movement**.

The earliest language you ever learned
was the feeling of yourself in space:

- The weight of your limbs
- The sway of your balance
- The texture of the earth beneath your hands and feet
- The way your body adjusted to surfaces, pressures, and gravity

You were a sensory being long before you became a thinking one. And when life attempts to fracture you—through injury, fear, or aging—it often does so by dulling that ancient language.

What Is the Sensory Body?

Your **sensory body** is not a metaphor.
It is your *lived experience* of:

- **Proprioception** – knowing where your body is without looking
- **Vestibular sense** – awareness of balance, tilt, and acceleration
- **Tactile feedback** – richness of touch: pressure, vibration, texture, temperature
- **Interoception** – internal sensing of heartbeat, breath rhythm, tension, hunger, calm

These systems are not luxuries.
They are them
Without them, you are a ghost inside yourself.

Movement Restores Sensory Richness

Natural Movement doesn't just train muscles.
It **re-awakens perception**.

- **Crawling** reestablishes ground contact and limb coordination.
- **Balancing** sharpens vestibular precision and micro-adjustments.
- **Carrying and lifting** recalibrate proprioceptive mapping under shifting loads.
- **Rolling, flowing, and vaulting** reactivate spatial orientation, tactile engagement, and dynamic stability.

Each movement isn't just a task.
It's a **conversation**.

- Each footfall against stone
- Each fingertip grazing bark
- Each sway across unstable ground

Every signal says:

"I am here.
I am whole.
I am part of this world."

The hiker's ability to recover from the fall, to sprint across uneven forest, to stand poised on the ridge—wasn't just about strength or stamina.

It was **sensory mastery**.

A body that knew itself deeply, trusted itself instinctively, and navigated the world—not as a stranger, but as a native son.

You Are Not a Pyramid—You Are a Web

In the traditional view, the brain controlled the body, muscles responded, and everything else was just support staff.

But you are not a pyramid.

You are a web.

A tensegrity of breath, tissue, nerve, and intention.

No one system is always in charge.

The leader is the one who listens best to the moment.

Practical Sensory Restoration Through Movement

Sensory System	Movement Practice
Proprioception	Blindfolded balance drills, barefoot locomotion across varied terrain
Vestibular	Dynamic balance work (logs, rails), rolling and inversion patterns
Tactile	Barefoot movement on textured surfaces, tree climbing, environmental contact

Sensory System	Movement Practice
Interoception	Breath-focused ground movement, slow-flow sessions emphasizing internal awareness

You do not rebuild the sensory body by thinking. You rebuild it by **moving through the world** with **attention** and **intention**.

You are not just your memories.
You are not just your ambitions.

You are the sum of what you've experienced— the way your body has carried you, the way your nerves have adapted, the way your senses have mapped the world.

Movement shapes identity.

Because every movement, conscious or unconscious, tells a story:

> "I can."
> "I can't."
> "I dare."
> "I fear."
> "I endure."
> "I grow."

Over time, those stories become belief systems.
And those belief systems become identity.

When movement is lost—through injury, trauma, illness, or aging—
the consequences aren't just physical.
They reach into the roots of self-perception:

"I'm fragile now."
"I can't trust my balance."
"I'm slow."
"I'm broken."
"I'm falling behind."

And these beliefs don't stay neatly contained within the gym or the doctor's office. They bleed into relationships, careers, creativity, and spirituality.

Movement loss becomes identity loss.

But the body is not static.
It listens.
It adapts.
It is always capable of rewriting the story.

- When you balance on unstable ground and trust your body to find its way, you proclaim: *"I am capable."*
- When you vault a low obstacle and land safely, you maintain: *"I am agile."*
- When you carry a heavy load across uneven terrain, you reaffirm: *"I am strong and resourceful."*

Movement is not just physical action.
It is an emotional message.
It is self-definition made visible and visceral.

The hiker did not reclaim his life by thinking his way into confidence.
He reclaimed it by moving his way back into belief.

Each crawl, each sprint, each roll, each climb—
not just tasks—
testaments.

Each one whispering:

"You are still here.
You are still powerful.
You are still becoming."

Practical Movement Practices for Identity Restoration

Identity Element	Movement Practice
Strength	Loaded carries over natural terrain
Agility	Vaults, ground flow sequences
Resilience	Controlled falls and recoveries (e.g., rolling patterns)
Exploration	Unstructured natural movement play (trees, rocks, rivers)

You are not separate from nature.
You are not separate from your body.

But modern life trains you to believe otherwise.

We are taught that thinking is better than feeling.
That productivity holds more value than presence.
That the body is an object to control or shape—
rather than a sacred link between self and world.

But when you move—really move—
that illusion begins to dissolve.

Movement and Belonging

When you crawl through earth and pine needles,
you remember where you came from.

When you balance across a fallen tree,
you reclaim the birthright of coordination and focus.

When you climb, swing, carry, run—
you stop feeling like a detached observer of life.
You become life.

Your nervous system.
Your senses.
Your breath.
Your feet on the ground—

They don't just produce fitness.
They produce belonging.

The hiker didn't just train to become stronger.
He trained to remember:

- That he was part of the land he walked on.
- That he was built for these challenges.
- That his breath and the wind were not enemies, but kin.
- That his body wasn't a machine to discipline, but a living expression of presence, reverence, and becoming.

The Physiology of Belonging

Pathway	Experience
Interoception	Feeling your heartbeat, breath, and gut states in real time—restoring inner awareness
Proprioception & Vestibular	Feeling your body move through space—restoring physical confidence and spatial trust
Tactile Input	Reconnecting with the world through touch—restoring immediacy and reality
Breath–Nervous System Feedback	Regulating emotional stability through intentional, breath-led movement

These systems aren't abstract.

They are the **physiological gateways** to being present, in the moment.

Movement as Devotion

Movement, when done with intention, becomes a practice of devotion:

To your body.
To the moment.
To the people who raised you.
To the landscapes that shaped you.
Until the day you are no longer here.

It becomes a prayer without words.
A sacred reminder:

"I was given this vessel.
I was given this breath.

I was given this one wild chance
to feel it all."

A Framework for Life—Training for Meaning, Not Just Metrics

You don't need **another app**.
You don't need another **quantified goalpost**.
You don't need to chase numbers until life itself feels like a spreadsheet.

You need an active practice—
a way to move, breathe, recover, and adapt—
that keeps you connected to life,
not separated by an obsession with performance.

The Five Pillars of Purposeful Training

Pillar	Focus	Example Practice
Vitality	Train your energy systems naturally	Sprint short bursts, hike long durations, vary outputs
Adaptability	Navigate different environments, surfaces, and challenges	Crawl, balance, climb, lift irregular objects
Resilience	Stress to grow—recover to integrate	Cycle intensity and rest; monitor HRV and breath
Presence	Cultivate internal awareness while moving	Flow with breath, move barefoot, walk mindfully
Belonging	Reconnect to body, nature, and others	Train outdoors, play, move with community

Practical Framework for a Week

Day	Focus	Examples
1	Dynamic effort	Sprint intervals + vault drills
2	Low-intensity exploration	Long hike with barefoot intervals
3	Strength & coordination	Carry heavy objects, integrate crawling patterns
4	Recovery emphasis	Breathwork, ground flow, mobility circuits
5	Playful variability	Unstructured movement in nature
6	Dynamic effort	Light climbing + loaded carries
7	Full recovery	Nature immersion, slow walk, breath-led awareness

Notice:

- No rigid zones
- No obsessive calorie counting
- No "punishment" sessions

Only movement as communication: **Challenge. Recovery. Awareness. Growth.**

Why This Works

Because this is how biology expects you to live:

- Bursts of intensity
- Periods of exploration
- Deep recovery
- Ongoing adaptation

It's how every resilient organism **survives**.
It's how every capable human **thrives**.

Metrics are snapshots.
But life is not a snapshot.
Life is a movement.

The hiker didn't master his body through perfect apps or rigid calendars.
He mastered it through:

Living.
Listening.
Adapting.
Trusting the cycles written in his blood, his nerves, his spirit.

And so can you.

You began this journey **sprinting for your life.**
You moved through fire.
You fell.
You adapted.
You recovered.

You mapped your energy systems.
You felt your senses awaken.
You rewired your nervous system.
You restored your trust.

But what you've truly done—
beneath the muscle, beneath the science—
is remember **who you are.**

You are **not fragile.**
You are **not broken.**
You are not a set of limitations waiting to be managed.

You are **capable.**
You are **adaptable.**
You are **alive.**

And in movement,
you have found not just a path forward—
but a way back.

> Back to your breath.
> Back to your power.
> Back to your body, your earth, your purpose.

You are not meant to shrink from the world.
You are meant to meet it—

Feet grounded
Eyes open
Heart steady

You are meant to **bend**, not break.
To **fall**, not fracture.
To **rise** again and again—stronger, not just in **muscle**,
but in **meaning**.

The Physiology of Purpose

Move like it matters.
Because inside you,
it always does.

Movement made the brain.
Movement refines the brain.
Movement preserves the brain.

Movement is awareness made real.
Awareness becomes action.
Action becomes survival.

Survival gives rise to recovery.
Recovery gives rise to adaptation.
Adaptation gives rise to freedom.

Freedom is the ability to meet the world—
not as you wish it were,
but as it is—
and move through it beautifully.

Across every stage of life—
you move to become who you are meant to be.

- Movement tests the body
- Movement reveals the soul
- Movement rebuilds trust
- Movement transcends aging
- Movement becomes a conversation between life and will

"I am still becoming."

This is no longer a story about fitness.
This is a story about remembering —
that the power to survive,
the power to adapt,
the power to grow —
has always lived inside you.

And all it ever wanted... was for you to move.

EPILOGUE

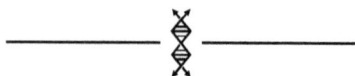

YOU WERE NEVER LOST

Maybe you didn't grow up climbing trees.
Maybe no one ever taught you how to crawl, vault, carry, or recover with purpose.
Maybe you spent more years sitting than sprinting.
Maybe you stopped trusting your body a long time ago.

But here's the truth:

You were never broken.
You were unpracticed in the language of your biology.

Every system inside you—
from mitochondria to muscle spindles,
from baroreceptors to breath rhythms—
has been waiting.

> Waiting for the signal.
> Waiting for the yes.
> Waiting for you to remember

that movement was never about performance.
It was about possibility.
It was about becoming.

You now understand: The body isn't a machine.
It's an orchestra—a symphony of systems, sounds, and
signals—
always ready to perform the song of survival, adaptation, and
joy.

And the conductor?
Is you.

So move.

Move like it matters.
Move with wonder.
Move with precision.
Move with joy.
Move with grief.
Move with love.
Move with whatever you have left.

But move.

Because every time you do,
you reclaim a piece of your power.

Every time you do,
you remind your body what it was built for.

Every time you do,
you say to the world—
and to yourself:

"I am here.
I am whole.
I am still becoming."

The Physiology of Purpose

You are the system.
You are the signal.
You are the reason.

And it's time—
finally—
to **move like it matters.**

THE PHYSIOLOGY OF PURPOSE – FULL REFERENCES

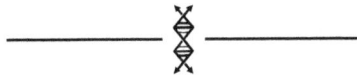

Lactate, Metabolism & Brain Signaling

- Brooks, G. A. (2021). Lactate in contemporary biology: A phoenix risen. The Journal of Physiology. https://doi.org/10.1113/JP279963

- Brooks, G. A. (2022a). Lactate as a fulcrum of metabolism. American Journal of Physiology–Endocrinology and Metabolism. https://doi.org/10.1152/ajpendo.00020.2022

- Brooks, G. A. (2022b). Tracing the lactate shuttle to the mitochondrial reticulum. Experimental & Molecular Medicine. https://doi.org/10.1038/s42255-021-00419-2

- Poole, D. C., et al. (2020). Anaerobic threshold: 50+ years of controversy. The Journal of Physiology. https://doi.org/10.1113/JP278930

- Hashimoto, T., et al. (2018). Maintained exercise-enhanced brain executive function related to cerebral lactate metabolism in men. The FASEB Journal. https://doi.org/10.1096/fj.201700381RR

- Wu, A., Lee, D., & Xiong, W.-C. (2023). Lactate metabolism, signaling, and function in brain development, synaptic plasticity, angiogenesis, and neurodegenerative diseases. International Journal of Molecular Sciences, 24(17), 13398. https://doi.org/10.3390/ijms241713398

- Wang, Y., Li, P., Xu, Y., Feng, L., Fang, Y., Song, G., Xu, L., Zhu, Z., Wang, W., Mei, Q., & Xie, M. (2024, November 28). Lactate metabolism and histone lactylation in the central nervous system disorders: Impacts and molecular mechanisms. Journal of Neuroinflammation, 21, Article 308. https://doi.org/10.1186/s12974-024-02975-4

- Riske, L. (2017). Lactate in the brain: An update. Therapeutic Advances in Psychopharmacology, 7(2), 85–89. https://doi.org/10.1177/2045125316675579

- Frontiers in Nutrition. (2022). Lactate is answerable for brain function. Frontiers in Nutrition, 9, Article 800901. https://doi.org/10.3389/fnut.2021.800901

- Morland, C., et al. (2017). Exercise induces cerebral angiogenesis via lactate receptor HCAR1. Nature Communications. https://doi.org/10.1038/s41467-017-00323-3

- El Hayek, L., et al. (2019). Lactate mediates exercise effects on learning and memory via SIRT1–BDNF signaling. Cell Metabolism. https://doi.org/10.1016/j.cmet.2019.04.015

- Bergersen, L. H. (2015). Lactate transport and signaling in the brain: Potential therapeutic targets and roles in body-brain interaction. Journal of Cerebral Blood Flow & Metabolism. https://doi.org/10.1038/jcbfm.2014.206

Motor Learning, Movement Coordination & Development

- Davids, K., Button, C., & Bennett, S. (2008). Dynamics of skill acquisition: A constraints-led approach. Human Kinetics.

- Gibson, J. J. (1979). The ecological approach to visual perception. Houghton Mifflin.

- Newell, K. M. (1986). Constraints on the development of coordination. In M. G. Wade & H. T. A. Whiting (Eds.), Motor development in children: Aspects of coordination and control (pp. 341–360). Martinus Nijhoff.

- Schmidt, R. A., & Lee, T. D. (2019). Motor learning and performance (6th ed.). Human Kinetics.

- Kolář, P. (2014). DNS: Principles of dynamic neuromuscular stabilization. Rehabilitation Prague School.

- Janda, V. (1983). Muscle function testing. Butterworths.

- Biotensegrity, Structural Integration, & Systems Theory

- Levin, S. M. (2002). The tensegrity-truss as a biomechanical model for the living body. Journal of Mechanics in Medicine and Biology, 2(3–4), 375–388. https://doi.org/10.1142/S021951940200047X

- Scarr, G. (2014). Biotensegrity: The structural basis of life. Handspring Publishing.
- Turvey, M. T., & Fonseca, S. (2014). The medium of haptic perception: A tensegrity hypothesis. Journal of Motor Behavior, 46(3), 143–187. https://doi.org/10.10 80/00222895.2013.798252

Stress, Recovery & HRV

- Lehrer, P. M., & Gevirtz, R. (2014). Heart rate variability biofeedback: How and why does it work? Frontiers in Psychology, 5, Article 756. https://doi.org/10.3389/ fpsyg.2014.00756
- Shaffer, F., & Ginsberg, J. P. (2017). An overview of heart rate variability metrics and norms. Frontiers in Public Health, 5, Article 258. https://doi.org/10.3389/ fpubh.2017.00258
- Thayer, J. F., & Lane, R. D. (2007). The role of vagal function in the risk for cardiovascular disease and mortality. Biological Psychology, 74(2), 224–242. https://doi.org/10.1016/j.biopsycho.2005.11.013

Neuroplasticity, Pain, Injury, & Recovery

- Grooms, D. R., & Myer, G. D. (2017). Upgraded hardware—What about the software? Brain updates for return to play following ACL reconstruction. Journal of Athletic Training, 52(6), 576–578. https:// doi.org/10.4085/1062-6050-52.2.09

- Moseley, G. L., & Butler, D. S. (2003). Explain Pain. Noigroup Publications.
- Sherrington, C. S. (1906). The Integrative Action of the Nervous System. Yale University Press.

Movement & Aging

- Fragala, M. S., Cadore, E. L., Dorgo, S., Izquierdo, M., Kraemer, W. J., Peterson, M. D., & Ryan, E. D. (2019). Resistance training for older adults: Position statement from the National Strength and Conditioning Association. Ageing Research Reviews, 51, 64–85. https://doi.org/10.1016/j.arr.2019.01.002
- Lexell, J. (1995). Human aging, muscle mass, and fiber type composition. The Journals of Gerontology Series A: Biological Sciences and Medical Sciences, 50A(Special Issue), 11–16. https://doi.org/10.1093/gerona/50A.Special_Issue.11
- Seidler, R. D., Bernard, J. A., Burutolu, T. B., Fling, B. W., Gordon, M. T., Gwin, J. T., Kwak, Y., & Lipps, D. B. (2010). Motor control and aging: Links to age-related brain structural, functional, and biochemical effects. Neuroscience & Biobehavioral Reviews, 34(5), 721–733. https://doi.org/10.1016/j.neubiorev.2009.10.005

Immunity & Movement

- Gleeson, M. (2007). Immune function in sport and exercise. Journal of Applied Physiology, 103(2),

693–699. https://doi.org/10.1152/japplphy-siol.00008.2007

- Nieman, D. C. (1994). Exercise, infection, and immunity. International Journal of Sports Medicine, 15(S3), S131–S141. https://doi.org/10.1055/s-2007-1021128

Natural Movement & Evolutionary Physiology

- Hébert, G. (1912). L'éducation physique par la méthode naturelle. Reprint editions.

- Kolb, B., & Whishaw, I. Q. (2001). An introduction to brain and behavior. Worth Publishers.

- Le Corre, E. (2019). The practice of natural movement. Victory Belt Publishing.

- Lieberman, D. E. (2013). The story of the human body: Evolution, health, and disease. Pantheon.

- Sapolsky, R. M. (2004). Why zebras don't get ulcers: The acclaimed guide to stress, stress-related diseases, and coping. Holt Paperbacks.

- Van Hooren, B., Fuller, J. T., Buckley, J. D., Miller, J. R., Sewell, K., Rao, G., & Barton, C. J. (2020). Is motorized treadmill running biomechanically comparable to overground running? A systematic review and meta-analysis of cross-over studies. Sports Medicine, 50, 785–813. https://doi.org/10.1007/s40279-019-01237-z

Author-Sourced and Perplexity-Aided Research

- The following references were curated by the author using personal research notes, professional literature, and insights aided by Perplexity's research platform.

- Author's research documents and notes from Move Because You Can (2023).

- Behm, D. G., & Sale, D. G. (1993). Intended rather than actual movement velocity determines velocity-specific training response.

- Davids, K., Button, C., & Bennett, S. (2012). An ecological dynamics approach to skill acquisition: Implications for development of talent in sport.

- Gibson, J. J. (1979). The Ecological Approach to Visual Perception. Houghton Mifflin.

- Kempermann, G., Kuhn, H. G., & Gage, F. H. (2010). Environmental enrichment, new neurons, and the neurobiology of individuality.

- La Scala Teixeira, C. V., Evangelista, A. L., Da Silva Grigoletto, M. E., et al. (2017). Effects of functional training on functional movement and muscular fitness in athletes.

- Proske, U., & Gandevia, S. C. (2012). The proprioceptive senses: Their roles in signaling body shape, body position and movement, and muscle force.

- Schleip, R., Findley, T. W., Chaitow, L., & Huijing, P. A. (2012). Fascia: The Tensional Network of the Human Body. Churchill Livingstone.

- Sherrington, C., Fairhall, N., Wallbank, G., et al. (2017). Exercise for preventing falls in older people living in the community. Cochrane Database of Systematic Reviews.

- Stergiou, N., & Decker, L. M. (2011). Human movement variability, nonlinear dynamics, and pathology: Is there a connection? Human Movement Science, 30(5), 869–888.

- van Praag, H., Kempermann, G., & Gage, F. H. (2000). Neural consequences of environmental enrichment. Nature Reviews Neuroscience, 1(3), 191–198.

- Wulf, G., & Lewthwaite, R. (2016). Optimizing performance through intrinsic motivation and attention for learning: The OPTIMAL theory of motor learning. Psychonomic Bulletin & Review, 23(5), 1382–1414.

MORE ACKNOWLEDGMENTS

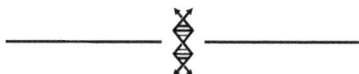

I want to extend my heartfelt thanks to Nicholas Cass and the entire team at Authors Unite for their dedication in bringing this book to life. Your commitment to thoughtful revision and design helped shape this project into something I'm truly proud of.

A special thank you to Lisa Krohn, whose attentive proofreading helped reveal the subtle gaps between what I was trying to convey and what the reader might actually perceive. Her curiosity, especially around the narrative elements woven throughout the text, led to important clarifications that ultimately made the story more cohesive and effective.

Finally, I'm deeply grateful to my editor, Michael Tizzano, for his steady hand in refining the manuscript. He preserved my voice while shaping the content into something more readable and accessible.

www.ingramcontent.com/pod-product-compliance
Lightning Source LLC
Chambersburg PA
CBHW062120020426
42335CB00013B/1031